Surgical Techniques for Prostate Cancer

Rakesh V. Khanna • Gennady Bratslavsky
Robert J. Stein

Editors

Surgical Techniques for Prostate Cancer

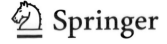 Springer

Editors
Rakesh V. Khanna
Department of Urology
SUNY Upstate Medical University
Syracuse, NY, USA

Gennady Bratslavsky
Department of Urology
SUNY Upstate Medical University
Syracuse, NY, USA

Robert J. Stein
Center for Robotic and Image
  Guided Surgery
Cleveland Clinic
Cleveland, OH, USA

ISBN 978-1-4939-1615-3   ISBN 978-1-4939-1616-0 (eBook)
DOI 10.1007/978-1-4939-1616-0
Springer New York Heidelberg Dordrecht London

Library of Congress Control Number: 2014950421

Springer is part of Springer Science+Business Media (www.springer.com)

Foreword

It gives me extreme pleasure to contribute this Foreword to an outstanding text about something near-and-dear to my heart: prostate cancer and surgery. Having been a student of prostate cancer and a radical prostatectomist for over 25 years, I am delighted to report that this book will not disappoint and will update us all on the ever-changing world of prostate cancer!

When I started my uro-oncology fellowship at Duke University in 1989, radical perineal prostatectomy was the most common prostate cancer operation, the nerve-sparing retropubic prostatectomy was still in its infancy, the first oral antiandrogen, flutamide, had just been FDA-approved and the PSA-Era had not even begun! For students and residents reading this, think about your future careers and imagine where we might be 25 years from now! But, let's ground ourselves in 2014 and take a look at surgical therapy. Fortunately, the anatomy, physiology, and embryology have not changed and Chap. 1 provides a very nice review of this important basic information essential for all students of the prostate.

In 2012, the United States Preventative Services Task Force (USPSTF) gave the PSA test a "D" rating for population-based screening. In 2013, the American Urological Association (AUA), called for every 2 year PSA testing only in men between the ages of 55 and 69. Because of these and other professional society policy changes, many practices have seen a decline in prostate biopsy, radical prostatectomy, and other surgical therapy as a result of this backlash against screening. So far, there is no solid documentation of a reverse stage migration, but I sense that there will be a growing use of surgical therapy for higher risk men in the near future. In addition, we are in the midst of an explosion of interest and use of active surveillance that is cutting into surgical volume, no pun intended! In the setting of active surveillance, TRUS Biopsy is more commonly performed and repeated. Chapter 2 provides a very complete review of contemporary prostate TRUS biopsy.

With regard to focal surgical therapy (i.e., focal cryotherapy and HIFU), it is unclear if this relatively new option will flourish in the future or remain a fringe treatment taking a back seat to active surveillance. Chapter 10 nicely covers the current state of the art regarding focal therapy. We are also on the heels of renewed interest in prostate MRI now that multi-parametric dynamic contrast enhanced techniques are proliferating. The biggest challenges now are for technique and reporting standardization, better training of specialized radiology providers, and clearer practice guidelines. However, it is possible and even probable that this may be a future game changer for better patient selection for surveillance vs. focal vs. radical surgical therapy. Chapter 3 provides a very nice and timely update.

As far as radical prostatectomy, the open vs. robotic debate continues and Chaps. 4–7 very expertly cover open, laparoscopic, robotic, and perineal approaches. We still have no available randomized controlled level I evidence to inform us. While I remain a fan of the retropubic open technique, the key message is experience, volume, care-pathways, and a skilled team for optimal outcomes. Patients should seek experienced providers and not focus so much on the robot or approach itself. We now know after more than 10 years that the robotic device is a tool and not the surgeon. It is marvelous technology and I applaud the fact that urologic surgeons were on the forefront; however, it does not substitute for experience and will not improve "The Trifecta" in and of itself. The robot era has made all of us, both open and robotic surgeons, better. It has made us better "students of the operation" and made us rethink all the steps to improve outcomes. For example, in my practice, the "competition" from the robot has taught me to try to make the smallest incision possible, to use liberal local anesthesia in the incision area, to use pre-op overactive bladder medications, and to provide better patient education about postoperative care and expectations. It is now all about improving short-term and long-term patient satisfaction. This has been wonderful for our patients and I thank the "robotic era" for that.

Prostate cryotherapy has seen a marked progression in technological advancement over the past 20 plus years. We are now on the fourth generation equipment combined with improved imaging and Chap. 9 provides a great review. Whether mp-MRI and MRI-directed prostate biopsy will allow more effective use of focal therapy remains to be seen in 2014. Total gland cryotherapy, while efficient and safe, is still hampered by collateral damage to the neurovascular bundles and unacceptability high rates of impotence limiting applicability for younger and potent men. High intensity focused ultrasound (HIFU) remains non-FDA approved and I hesitate to speculate on its future. Brachytherapy remains a very viable option and is one of the best local therapies for potency preservation. Chapter 8 is devoted to prostate brachytherapy.

Whatever surgical therapy for prostate cancer is chosen, it is critical for surgeons not to operate in a vacuum. In other words, patients benefit from a multidisciplinary approach whether it is low risk localized disease to locally advanced high risk disease. At my institution, we are celebrating 10 years of conducting a true multi-D clinic where patients are seen by a surgeon, a radiation oncologist, and a medical oncologist. In our published experience from 2005 to 2009 with over 700 patients, 51 % of patients chose radical prostatectomy. In my opinion, these men were the most gratifying to operate on since they had chosen surgical therapy only after a very complete education about all the options. In addition, surgical therapy does not obviously cure all men and it is right to ensure these men already have a relationship with other team specialists beforehand.

As far as neoadjuvant and adjuvant therapy to surgery, there is much still to be learned. Harking back to 20 years ago, neoadjuvant hormonal therapy to radical prostatectomy was all the rage. Unfortunately, surgical "down-staging" did not come to pass and traditional HT before RP is now only occasionally used for technical down-sizing. However, with six novel therapeutic agents FDA-approved for advanced prostate cancer between 2010 and 2013, the concept of neoadjuvant therapy is being re-visited. In the future, drugs like Abiraterone or Enzalutamide may see a common use in this presurgical or postsurgical setting. As we go to press, exciting data suggests that Docetaxel systemic chemotherapy given along with hormonal therapy to men with newly diagnosed M1 prostate cancer extended survival by over 1 year. This is game-changing data. I wonder if we will be operating on men with metastatic disease in the future—particularly ones with minimal metastatic disease who have a robust initial response to systemic therapy?

In summary, Doctors Rakesh V. Khanna, Gennady Bratslavsky, and Robert J. Stein who edited this text must be congratulated for organizing a stellar summary. I also want to commend all the individual authors and co-authors for their hard work in summarizing each chapter in a concise and up-to-date manner. Finally, to my fellow prostate cancer students, scholars, and surgeons, I would like to say how fortunate we all are to be working in such a stimulating area and for having the privilege of caring for our patients. I would like to dedicate this Foreword to both the civilian and military patients who I have had to honor and pleasure to care for during my career. I hope that I will continue to have this opportunity and honor for many years to come.

Durham, NC, USA   Judd W. Moul, M.D., F.A.C.S.
                                                    Division of Urology, Department of Surgery
                                                        Duke Cancer Institute, Duke University

Preface

Prostate cancer is the most common cancer in men after skin cancer and is the second leading cause of cancer death. Today most prostate cancers arise as clinically nonpalpable disease detected through PSA screening at a time when patients often have no identifiable symptoms.

This is at the heart of treatment for localized prostate cancer. We take patients, many of whom are asymptomatic, and expose them to the risks of treatment not limited just to erectile dysfunction or incontinence but also including fistula, bleeding, and stricture disease, just to name a few.

This is further amplified with the controversies in PSA screening. It is important that we adequately council our patients on the risks and benefits of getting screened and in those who are found to have prostate cancer on the available treatment options.

It was in this regard that this manuscript was written. It is not the goal of this manuscript to advise which patients should be treated. Instead, for those who are selected to be treated, it is the aim of this manuscript to provide a manual to the Urologist specializing in prostate cancer treatment, starting with the time of diagnosis, proceeding to various treatment options as well as techniques to optimize outcomes.

For the Urologist, numerous surgical approaches are available to treat patients, including Surgery, Radiation therapy (Brachytherapy), and Focal therapy.

We begin by detailing prostate anatomy. We then proceed with explaining optimal prostate biopsy techniques (both ultrasound guided as well as MRI fusion). We then explore the various surgical techniques including open, laparoscopic, robotic, and perineal prostatectomy. Urologists also often work with colleagues in Radiation Oncology performing brachytherapy and a chapter has also been included on this technique as well. In addition we also discuss cryotherapy and conclude with future directions in prostate cancer treatment.

This is a lot to cover. When we started this project, there was no concise manuscript covering prostate cancer surgery written for urologists. For the urologists specializing in prostate cancer treatment, we hope this manuscript will fill this need.

We are very excited to have an international list of contributors. They are experts in the field. Going through the chapters, we have learned a lot from reading their work—we think the reader will too.

To the reader, please let us know your comments, including topics that you would like to have covered in future editions. What can we do in the future to make this manuscript better—remember it was written for you!

Hoping that this manuscript makes your practice a little easier … and more importantly, hoping for the day we find a cure for prostate cancer and manuals such as these are no longer needed…

Syracuse, NY, USA   Rakesh V. Khanna, M.D.
Syracuse, NY, USA   Gennady Bratslavsky, M.D.
Cleveland, OH, USA   Robert J. Stein, M.D.

Acknowledgements

I wish to thank the Almighty for providing me the opportunity and ability to develop this manuscript.

I wish to thank all the authors who took time out of their busy schedules to contribute to this edition. A special thanks also goes to Connie Walsh who put all the chapters together into the beautiful volume you hold in front of you.

This work is dedicated with respect to my wonderful wife, parents, and family. This work would not have been possible were it not for their constant support and encouragement.

Rakesh V. Khanna

Contents

Contributors

Gennady Bratslavsky, M.D. Department of Urology, SUNY Upstate Medical University, Syracuse, NY, USA

Timothy Byler, M.D. Department of Urology, SUNY Upstate Medical University, Syracuse, NY, USA

Jay P. Ciezki, M.D. Department of Radiation Oncology, Taussig Cancer Institute, Cleveland Clinic Foundation, Cleveland, OH, USA

Forrestall O. Dorsett Jr., M.D., M.B.A. General Surgery, SUNY Upstate University Hospital, Syracuse, NY, USA

Bertrand D. Guillonneau, M.D., Ph.D., Dr. h.c. Department of Urology, Diaconesses-Croix St. Simon Hospital, Paris, France

J. Stephen Jones, M.D. Glickman Urological and Kidney Institute, Cleveland Clinic Foundation, Cleveland, OH, USA

Rakesh V. Khanna, M.D. Department of Urology, SUNY Upstate Medical University, Syracuse, NY, USA

Nikhil Khattar, M.B.B.S., M.S., M.Ch. (Urol.) Department of Urology, PGIMER and Dr Ram Manohar Lohia Hospital, New Delhi, India

Eric A. Klein, M.D. Glickman Urological and Kidney Institute, Cleveland Clinic Foundation, Cleveland, OH, USA

Joseph C. Klink, M.D. Glickman Urological and Kidney Institute, Center for Urologic Oncology, Cleveland Clinic Foundation, Cleveland, OH, USA

Michael C. Lee, M.D. Harvard Vanguard Medical Associates, An Affiliate of Atrius Health, Boston, MA, USA

Guilherme Maia, M.D. Department of Urology, Diaconesses-Croix St. Simon Hospital, Paris, France

Judd W. Moul, M.D. Division of Urology, Department of Surgery Duke Cancer Institute, Duke University, Durham, NC, USA

Rishi Nayyar, M.S., M.Ch., F.M.A.S. Department of Urology, PGIMER and Dr Ram Manohar Lohia Hospital, New Delhi, India

Imad Nsouli, M.D. Department of Urology, SUNY, Upstate Medical University, Syracuse, NY, USA

Urology Division, Surgery Department, VA Medical Center, Syracuse, NY, USA

Julio M. Pow-Sang, M.D. Department of Genitourinary, Division of Oncology, H. Lee Moffitt Cancer Center and Research Institute, Tampa, FL, USA

Rajeev Sood, M.B.B.S., M.S. (Surg.), M.Ch. (Urol.) Department of Urology, Dr Ram Manohar Lohia Hospital and PGI MER PGIMER and Dr Ram Manohar Lohia Hospital, New Delhi, India

Robert J. Stein, M.D. Center for Robotic and Image Guided Surgery, Glickman Urological and Kidney Institute, Cleveland Clinic, Cleveland, OH, USA

Kevin L. Stephans, M.D. Department of Radiation Oncology, Taussig Cancer Institute, Cleveland Clinic Foundation, Cleveland, OH, USA

Itay Sternberg, M.D. Department of Urology, Memorial Sloan Kettering Cancer Center, New York, NY, USA

Einar F. Sverrisson, M.D. Department of Genitourinary, Division of Oncology, H. Lee Moffitt Cancer Center and Research Institute, Tampa, FL, USA

Abdelkarim Touijer, M.D. Department of Urology, Memorial Sloan Kettering Cancer Center, New York, NY, USA

Oscar M. Valderrama, M.D. Department of Genitourinary, Division of Oncology, H. Lee Moffitt Cancer Center and Research Institute, Tampa, FL, USA

Srinivas Vourganti, M.D. State University of New York, Upstate Medical University, Syracuse, NY, USA

Matthew C. Ward, M.D. Department of Radiation Oncology, Taussig Cancer Institute, Cleveland Clinic Foundation, Cleveland, OH, USA

Andrij R. Wojtowycz, M.D. Diagnostic Division, Department of Radiology, SUNY Upstate Medical University, Syracuse, NY, USA

Essentials of the Human Prostate

Forrestall O. Dorsett Jr.

Overview

In this chapter we will review the development, anatomy, and physiology of the prostate and seminal vesicles.

The prostate gland is a single organ that encircles the urethra. It is approximately 20 g in volume, 3 cm in length, 4 cm wide, and 2 cm in depth. Some things can cause these dimensions to vary. Of particular clinical significance is benign prostatic hyperplasia (BPH) which can develop as men age and lead to urinary obstruction. This condition can then gradually lead to upper tract pathology as well.

Anatomically the prostate is found posterior to the pubic symphysis, superior to the perineal membrane, inferior to the bladder, and anterior to the rectum (Fig. 1.1). The gland is supported anteriorly by the pubo-prostatic ligaments and inferiorly by the external urethral sphincter and perineal membrane.

Anatomy

The prostate can be separated into four regions; anterior, peripheral, central, and transitional zones (Fig. 1.2). These zones are important in that they each can be the site of distinct pathology. The anterior fibromuscular zone which represents 30 % of the prostate mass contains virtually no glandular elements and is primarily smooth muscle. The peripheral zone is the largest zone, comprising 75 % of prostate glandular elements. It is of significant clinical importance as it is the primary site of prostatic carcinomas. The central zone has roughly 20–25 % of prostate glandular elements and surrounds ejaculatory ducts while the transitional zone contains up to 5 % of prostate glandular elements, is the site of BPH, and represents approximately 15–30 % of prostate volume.

The prostate is the only solid organ in the pelvis and is typically easily located on digital rectal exam (DRE) especially when enlarged. It has been classically described as being about the size of a walnut with a texture not unlike the tip of the nose when palpated. It is oriented with its base angled posteriorly toward the bladder neck and its apex is angled anteriorly in continuity with the urethra. At the apex of the prostate we have the formation of the striated external urethral sphincter (Fig. 1.3). This sphincter is a vertically oriented tubular sheath that surrounds the membranous urethra and prostate. The gland is also suspended by the pubo-rectal

F.O. Dorsett Jr., M.D., M.B.A. (✉)
General Surgery, SUNY Upstate University Hospital,
Syracuse, NY, USA

883 Crestwell Circle, Atlanta, GA 30331, USA
e-mail: Fordor27@hotmail.com

R.V. Khanna et al. (eds.), *Surgical Techniques for Prostate Cancer*,
DOI 10.1007/978-1-4939-1616-0_1, © Springer Science+Business Media New York 2015

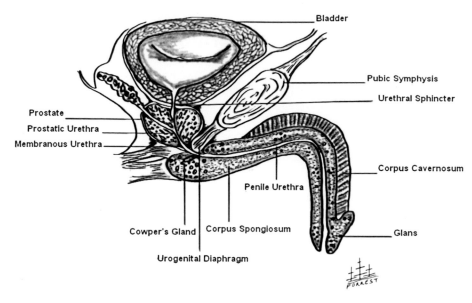

Fig. 1.1 Prostate and its anatomic relationships. All illustrations by Forrestall O. Dorsett Jr.

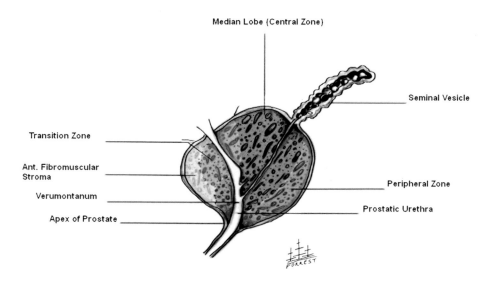

Fig. 1.2 Zones of the prostate

portion of the levator ani muscle (Fig. 1.4). The prostate possesses an outer capsule which is made up of collagen, smooth muscle, and elastin. The longitudinal fibers of the detrusor muscle mesh with the fibro-muscular tissue of the capsule. While contributing to the rubbery external texture of the prostate and some protective benefit, the capsule also serves as scaffolding for adjacent support structures besides the levator ani. Additional support is provided by three distinct yet intertwining layers of fascia found on the anterior, lateral, and posterior aspects of the prostate. The anterior and antero-lateral fascia is in direct continuity of the capsule. This is where the deep dorsal vein of the penis and its tributaries are found. Laterally the levator fascia fuses with the anterior and antero-lateral fascia. The recto-vesical or Denonvilliers fascia is a connective tissue layer located between

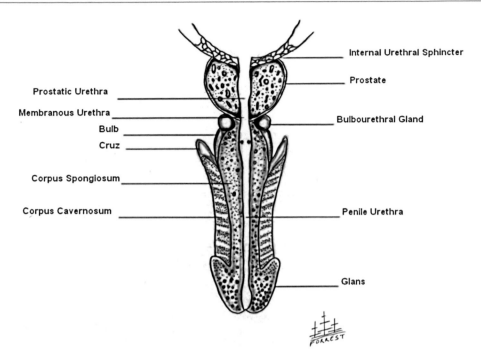

Fig. 1.3 Coronal view of penis and prostate

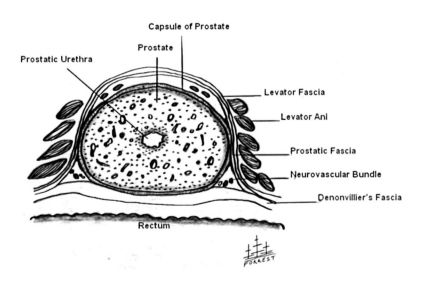

Fig. 1.4 Axial view of prostate showing muscle fibers of levator ani

the anterior wall of the rectum and posterior aspect of the prostate. This fascial layer covers the prostate and seminal vesicles posteriorly and extends caudally to terminate as a fibrous plate just below the urethra at the level of the external urethral sphincter near the apex of the prostate. This median fibrous plate or raphe has a distal extension to the level of the central tendon of the perineum.

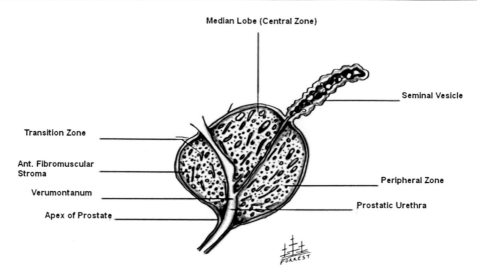

Fig. 1.5 Sagittal cross-section of prostate

Seminal Vesicles

The seminal vesicles are two saccular glands that pair with its corresponding ductus to form the ejaculatory ducts that enter into the prostate. The seminal vesicles are located superior to the prostate under the base of the bladder and are approximately 6 cm in length (Fig. 1.5). Seminal vesicles are derived from the wolffian ducts through testosterone stimulation. Together with the prostate the seminal vesicles create seminal fluid that facilitates sperm transport for fertilization.

Gland General Composition

Epithelial cells: Basal, Intermediate, Columnar secretory, Neuroendocrine

Stromal cells: Smooth muscle, Fibroblast, Endothelial

Tissue matrix: Extracellular matrix, Basement membrane, Connective tissue, Glycosaminoglycans, Cytomatrix, Nuclear matrix

Prostate Zones

Anterior fibromuscular: 30 % of prostate mass, no glandular elements, smooth muscle

Peripheral: Largest zone, 75 % of prostate glandular elements, site of carcinomas

Central: 25 % of prostate glandular elements; surrounds ejaculatory ducts

Transitional: 5 % of prostate glandular elements, site of BPH, 15–30 % of prostate volume

Embryology

The prostate is a derivative of the primitive endoderm. This tubular structure differentiates into the foregut, midgut, and hindgut as well as a distal structure called the cloaca. The cloaca then divides into separate urinary and digestive outlets by the urorectal septum. The ventral urinary compartment is called the primitive urogenital sinus, which further segments into the urinary bladder at its cranial end and the urethra at its caudal terminus.

Development of the prostate is actually induced by the primitive prostatic urethra. This occurs when epithelial buds in the prostatic segment of the urethra extend into the surrounding mesenchyme at around week 10 of gestation. This epithelial budding is strictly androgen-dependent and represents the first events in prostate development. At around week 12 the distinct lobes of the prostate can be distinguished.

The wolffian ducts develop into the seminal vesicles, epididymis, vas deferens, ampulla, and ejaculatory duct. The developmental growth of this group of glands is stimulated by fetal testosterone and not dihydrotestosterone.

Innervation

The prostate has autonomic input from both parasympathetic and sympathetic sources. Innervations of the prostate arise from the pelvic plexuses formed by the parasympathetic, visceral, efferent, and preganglionic fibers from the sacral levels S2–S4. These sacral levels also incidentally are directly related to erectile function which is an immense consideration during prostatic surgery where nerve sparing remains a viable option. The sympathetic fibers arise from the thoraco-lumbar levels (L1–L2). The pelvic plexus is located beside the rectum approximately 7 cm from the anal verge, with its midpoint located at the level of the tips of the seminal vesicles (Fig. 1.6). The sympathetic and parasympathetic fibers that come from the pelvic plexuses travel to the prostate via the cavernous nerves. The cavernous nerves run posterolateral to the prostate in the lateral prostatic fascia. The parasympathetic nerves end at the acini and lead to prostatic secretion. This is demonstrated by the use of muscarinic cholinergic agonists which has a marked effect on increasing prostatic secretion. The sympathetic nerves lead to contraction of the smooth muscle of the capsule and the stroma.

Another important nerve related to the prostate is the pudendal nerve. The pudendal nerve is the major nerve supply leading to somatic innervations of the striated sphincter and the levator ani. The preprostatic sphincter and the bladder neck (or internal sphincter) is under alpha-adrenergic control. The α_{1A} receptor appears to be linked to smooth muscle contraction of the prostate. This is of clinical importance because of the use of selective α_1-adrenergic antagonists to alleviate bladder outlet obstruction secondary to BPH.

Arterial Supply

The main arterial supply to the prostate comes from the inferior vesical artery (IVA) which itself stems from the anterior division of the internal iliac artery. This artery also supplies the base of the bladder and distal ureters. The IVA branches into the urethral artery and the capsular artery.

The urethral artery enters the prostate-vesical junction postero-laterally and travels inward perpendicular to the urethra toward the bladder neck at approximately the 5 o'clock and 7 o'clock meridian. The urethral artery then turns caudally and parallel to the urethra to supply the transition zone. This artery is the main arterial supply for the adenomas in BPH.

The capsular artery runs postero-lateral to the prostate with the cavernous nerves (Fig. 1.7). This artery enters the prostate at right angles to supply the glandular tissue.

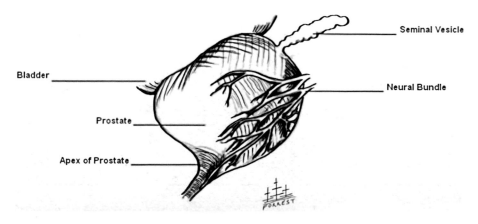

Fig. 1.6 Prostate demonstrating innervation

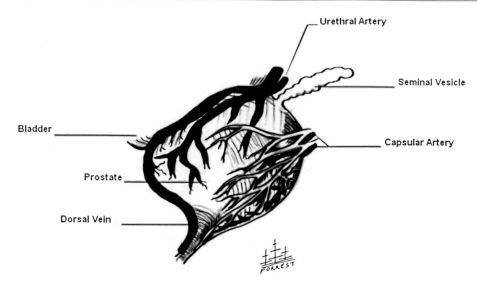

Fig. 1.7 Prostate demonstrating innervation

The prostatic vessels and the autonomic innervations run between the layers of the lateral prostatic fascia and the prostate.

The arterial blood supply to the seminal vessels and ductus deferens comes from the deferential artery or artery of the ductus, a branch from the superior vesical artery.

Venous Drainage

Venous drainage of the prostate begins with the deep dorsal vein (Fig. 1.7). This is a continuation of the vein that is often plainly visible on the dorsal surface of the penis. After this vein leaves the penis beneath the Buck fascia and under the pubic arch, it passes antero-superior to the perineal membrane. The vein then divides into the superficial, right and left branches.

The superficial branch travels between the pubo-prostatic ligaments and lies on top of the prostate and bladder neck. The superficial branch is outside the anterior prostatic fascia in the retropubic fat and pierces the fascia to drain into the dorsal venous complex. The common trunk of the dorsal venous complex and the lateral venous plexuses are covered by the anterior prostatic fascia and the endopelvic fascia. The lateral plexuses travel postero-laterally and communicate with the pudendal, obturator, and vesical plexus.

These veins then communicate with the internal iliac vein.

Lymphatic Drainage

The lymphatic drainage of the prostate primarily drains to the obturator and the internal iliac lymphatic channels. There is also lymphatic communication with the external iliac, presacral, and the para-aortic lymph nodes.

Summary

Knowledge of prostatic anatomy is integral for effective diagnosis and treatment of prostate cancer. A sensible approach to surgical management depends on understanding the extent of disease in addition to familiarity with anatomic landmarks.

Suggested Reading

Anatomy: Campbell-Walsh Urology text, Alan J. Wein, MD, PhD(hon), Louis R. Kavoussi, MD, Andrew C. Novick, MD, Alan W. Partin, MD, PhD and Craig A. Peters, MD, FACS, FAAP

Embriology: http://www.ncbi.nlm.nih.gov/pmc/articles/PMC3071422/

http://onlinelibrary.wiley.com/doi/10.1111/j.1432-0436.2008.00303.x/full

Transrectal Ultrasound-Guided Prostate Biopsy

2

Michael C. Lee and J. Stephen Jones

Abbreviations

ASAP   Atypical small acinar proliferation
AUA   American Urological Association
DRE   Digital rectal exam
ERSPC   European Randomized Study of Screening for Prostate Cancer
HGPIN   High-grade prostatic intraepithelial neoplasia
IPSS   International Prostate Symptom Score
PSA   Prostate-specific antigen
RCTs   Randomized control trials
SHIM   Sexual Health Inventory for Men
TRUS   Transrectal ultrasound

Introduction

Astraldi first described transrectal prostate biopsy in 1937 through a digitally guided approach [1]. A major innovation in the late 1980s was incorporating transrectal ultrasound (TRUS) with prostate biopsy, taking TRUS beyond static prostatic imaging. Hodge et al. demonstrated the use of TRUS to guide biopsies in a directed fashion using six evenly distributed biopsies across the parasagittal plane [2]. Instead of targeting palpable masses or hypoechoic lesions, the application of random biopsies has increased the detection of early stage prostate cancer and has contributed to the stage migration of prostate cancer present today. The topic continues to evolve today and this chapter looks to highlight the applications and techniques as well as controversies and innovations within the field of prostate biopsy.

Indications

TRUS-directed prostate needle biopsy is the gold standard for the diagnosis of prostate cancer. Traditional indications for prostate biopsy arise from prostate cancer screening and include abnormal digital rectal exam (DRE) or abnormal prostate-specific antigen (PSA). Prostate cancer screening has become a controversial topic [3] and is out of the scope of this chapter. The American Urological Association (AUA) 2013 Prostate Cancer Detection Guidelines states "There is no PSA level below which a man can be informed that prostate cancer does not exist." Furthermore, "the Panel believes that the urologist should consider factors that lead to an increased PSA including prostate volume, age, and inflammation rather

M.C. Lee, M.D. (✉)
Harvard Vanguard Medical Associates, An Affiliate of Atrius Health, 133 Brookline Avenue, Boston, MA 02215, USA
e-mail: michaelc_lee@atriushealth.org

J.S. Jones, M.D.
Glickman Urological and Kidney Institute, Cleveland Clinic Foundation, Cleveland, OH, USA

R.V. Khanna et al. (eds.), *Surgical Techniques for Prostate Cancer*,
DOI 10.1007/978-1-4939-1616-0_2, © Springer Science+Business Media New York 2015

Needle Path

The transrectal approach is most common in prostate biopsy and is the main focus of the chapter. Nevertheless, two other needle paths deserve mention, (1) transurethral and (2) transperineal. Historically, transurethral prostate biopsy was thought to better sample the transition zone but the current application is extremely limited [24]. Transperineal biopsy offers an approach to patients without a rectum, but also has gained favor in certain locations due to the potential to more readily biopsy the anterior prostate. With the rise of brachytherapy, the development of template-guided biopsies, and the avoidance of a transrectal approach due to multi-drug resistant *E. coli*, this approach may be seen more frequently. The diagnostic yield of transperineal biopsy versus transrectal biopsy has been varied with the only randomized, prospective trial to date demonstrating no differences of yield or complications between the groups [25]. Most transperineal biopsies are performed under general or regional anesthesia, which has limited adoption of this approach in many locales.

Probe Type

The type of ultrasonography probe appears to play a role in the detection of prostate cancer in transrectal biopsy. End-fire TRUS probe is superior in both initial and repeat prostate biopsy compared to side-fire probes [26, 27]. The ability of the end-fire probe to access high-yield areas such as the lateral zone, anterior tissue, and apex may explain the higher cancer detection rates. Nevertheless, armed with the knowledge that the anterior prostate should be sampled, it has been demonstrated that equivalent detection rates may be achieved with the side fire probe if technique is optimized [28].

Number of Cores

Prostate biopsy was initially guided by digital-directed sampling of palpable nodules or ultrasound identification of suspicious lesions.

The cancer detection rate was then enhanced with the description of a sextant biopsy scheme that sample one core bilaterally from the base, mid, and apex [2]. Currently, the sextant scheme has been shown to be woefully inadequate for routine prostate biopsy for prostate cancer detection. The predominance of prostate cancer in the peripheral zone suggests under sampling of sextant biopsy and may explain false negative results. Extended biopsy protocols including 8–13 cores significantly enhanced the prostate cancer detection rate to upwards of 40 % compared sextant schemes (26 %) [29]. A large, multi-institutional study of community urologist involving 2,299 patients undergoing 12-core biopsy, overall cancer detection rate was 44 %, which is similar to the results of most academic single-center studies [30]. We recommend a 12–14 core extended-biopsy strategy for patient undergoing initial prostate biopsy, preferring to add two "extreme apical" cores based on our findings that these often identify unique cancers missed on the traditional 12 cores [31].

Saturation biopsies (defined today has minimum 20 transrectal cores taken at biopsy) were initially described in men with previous negative biopsies [32]. We have demonstrated that this is well tolerated under local anesthesia in the office setting thus reducing risk, time, and cost of using the operating room [33]. In our experience of over 1,000 saturation biopsies, we have not had increased complications compared to extended biopsy schemes [34]. By contrast, there is no role for transrectal saturation biopsy as initial prostate biopsy as cancer detection rates do not differ significantly from extended biopsy schemes even when stratified across PSA ranges [34].

Apical Biopsy

Apical biopsies are essential because of the high prevalence of cancers in this location, particularly anteriorly. In a true false negative biopsy, the anterior apical location is the most likely site of cancer missed [30]. The difficulty lies in accessibility especially for side-fire probes and patient pain during biopsy of the apex. We have reported that apical biopsy intolerance is not due to prostatic pain but is actually based on anal pain from sensory pain fibers below the dentate line of the rectum [35]. A rectal sensation test may avoid this pain by repositioning the needle about the dentate line, reaching an asensate area. Simply performing this maneuver may miss adequate apical biopsy by targeting the mid-gland. Aiming the probe handle craniodorsally pulls the rectal mucosa caudally, thus allowing painless apical biopsy.

Complications

Minor complications include bleeding, vasovagal response, and painful urination requiring analgesics. Bleeding in the form of hematuria, hematospermia, and hematochezia occur in 5.1–89 %, 12.5–80 %, and 1.3–59 % of patients, respectively [36–38]. Traditionally, aspirin and thrombolytics have been held 5–7 days prior to biopsy. There has been no correlation of previous aspirin use to the post-biopsy risk of bleeding [37]. Hematospermia may persist up to 4–6 weeks after biopsy, may cause patient distress but is of minimal clinical importance. Hematochezia can usually be controlled with direct pressure from the ultrasound probe or digitally. Persistent rectal bleeding rarely may require anoscopic intervention. A vasovagal response may be seen in 1.4–5.3 % of patients as a result of anxiety and discomfort [36].

Major complications have been reported at 0.6–2.5 % [30, 33–35]. In the absence of hematuria, urinary retention requiring catheterization occurs in 0.2–0.8 % of men [37, 39]. By contrast, this rate is approximately 10 % in reports of transperineal mapping biopsy, probably due to the requirement of general anesthesia. Significantly enlarged glands and severe lower urinary tract symptoms correlate to a higher risk of urinary retention [36, 37]. Clot retention requiring catheterization and irrigation occurs in 0.4–0.7 % [37, 39]. Post-biopsy infections are usually limited to symptomatic UTIs and low-grade fevers; however, rare cases of mortality from urosepsis have occurred. In this era with prophylactic antibiotics, the risk of urosepsis requiring hospitalization is 1.2–3.5 % [36–39]. The presence of quinolone-resistant bacteria is now upward of 30 % in men undergoing

biopsy [40], which may explain recent rise in urosepsis rates [41].

Cleveland Clinic identified and reported significantly increased infection rates in 2010 based on increasing fluoroquinolone resistance in patients who developed sepsis. We approached this in multidisciplinary fashion through collaboration with our colleagues specializing in infectious diseases. Through analysis of resistance patterns we added 1.5 mg/kg of intramuscular gentamicin for standard patients to the single dose ciprofloxacin. Based on the need for 24 h coverage, we switched the fluoroquinolone to levafloxacin 750 mg. In our non-published analysis of all patients called directly to identify infections, we now have the infection rate back down to 1.5 %.

Long-term complications including voiding dysfunction and erectile dysfunction have been described. Utilization of saturation biopsy demonstrated significant impairment of voiding as measured by the International Prostate Symptom Score (IPSS) at 3 months post-biopsy [42]. The same study demonstrated transient impairment of erectile function as measured by the International Index of Erectile Function [42]. As active surveillance has become a popular treatment modality for prostate cancer, the frequency of prostate biopsy in an individual may rise. The number of biopsies has been associated with decreasing Sexual Health Inventory for Men (SHIM) score though the same study failed to correlation between biopsy number and IPSS score [43].

Controversies

Repeat Biopsy Protocols

The approach to repeat biopsy after negative initial prostate biopsy is controversial. A 10–30 % cancer detection rate on repeat biopsy has been recognized. Transrectal saturation biopsy has been strongly advocated in the repeat biopsy setting [44]. We recently demonstrated saturation prostate biopsy had a statistically significant higher detection rate when compared to extended prostate biopsy at first repeat biopsy ($n = 1,462$, 33 % vs. 22.4 %, $p < 0.0001$), the difference persisted in patients diagnosed initially with truly benign findings, as well as HGPIN and ASAP [45]. Within this population, insignificant cancer (defined Gleason score <7, positive cores ≤3 and maximum percentage involvement of cancer in any positive core ≤50 %) was detected in 38.3 % patients with positive biopsy [45]. There was not a significant difference in the identification of clinically insignificant cancer between saturation and extended biopsy, although we believe there is a trend in that direction. We originally used a 24-core transrectal template with cores concentrated laterally and apically based on the preponderance of cancer in these locations. Based on our experience with site-specific labeling, the lateral sectors were the site of all unique tumors. As a result, we reduced sampling from two cores to one core per medial sector (mid-gland and base), resulting in a 20-core template for patients undergoing repeat biopsy [46].

Multiple Negative Biopsies

The chance of prostate cancer detection drops with more repeat biopsies. Multiple negative biopsies complicate the situation and raise the question whether there is a reasonable time point to stop the biopsy cascade. The European Randomized Study of Screening for Prostate Cancer (ERSPC) demonstrated sequentially lower rates of prostate cancer detected on repeat biopsy 1, 2, 3, and 4 with rates of 22 %, 10 %, 5 %, and 4 % respectively, with improved tumor characteristics (lower grade, stage, and volume) in the repeat biopsy 3 and 4 population [47]. The incidence of low-grade prostate cancer is 62 % in men with two negative previous biopsies [48]. We have shown that patients who had a second negative biopsy that was performed as a transrectal saturation biopsy have an exceedingly low likelihood of being diagnosed with significant prostate cancer in the future, so performing serial biopsy should be avoided without compelling reasons such as rapidly rising PSA or new findings of abnormal DRE [49]. Our opinion is in men with two previous negative biopsies, the indication to pursue additional biopsies is rare and reserved in men with high-risk indicators such as ASAP

and multifocal HGPIN. In the latter setting we recommend the protocol of Lepor and Taneja in performing delayed interval biopsy approximately every 3 years in men healthy enough to have treatment of prostate cancer [4, 49].

Future Directions

While the use of TRUS has significantly impacted prostate biopsy, TRUS-guided biopsies have limitations. The grayscale of TRUS is unreliable in differentiating normal prostate gland from cancerous tissue. Furthermore, the freehand technique is challenging and subjective, limiting the effect of described templates. Critics of TRUS cite this diagnosis and localization uncertainty as a barrier in the field. Current technologies in development include tracking systems, MRI-fused TRUS biopsy, and robotic systems [50]. Tracking systems like Artemis and TargetScan show the user the location of the probe in the image space while using traditional freehand manipulation of the probe through special navigation software, although their benefit remains hypothetical and not supported by the literature at this point in time. MRI-fused TRUS biopsy register pre-acquired MRI images to TRUS at the beginning of the procedure, thus allowing cancer suspicious regions on MRI to be easier targeted on TRUS biopsy. Robotics offer the opportunity to track the probe but may also facilitate automated needle targeting. Such technologies are preliminary and not the standard of care and critics would argue that the prostate is a mobile organ that changes in real-time with respirations, probe movements, operating table position, and multiple passes of the biopsy needle.

References

1. Astraldi A. Diagnosis of cancer of the prostate: biopsy by rectal route. Urol Cutaneous Rev. 1937;41:421.
2. Hodge KK, McNeal JK, Terris MK. Random systematic versus directed ultrasound guided transrectal core biopsies of the prostate. J Urol. 1989;142:71–4.
3. Moyer VA, et al. Screening for prostate cancer: U.S. Preventive Service Task Force Recommendation Statement. Ann Intern Med. 2012;157(2):120–34.

4. Lee MC, Moussa AS, Yu C, et al. Multifocal high grade prostatic intraepithelial neoplasia is a risk factor for subsequent prostate cancer. J Urol. 2010;184(5): 1958–62.

5. Abouassaly R, Tan N, Moussa A, et al. Risk of prostate cancer after diagnosis of atypical glands suspicious for carcinoma on saturation and traditional biopsies. J Urol. 2008;180(3):911–4.

6. Wolf JS, Bennett CJ, Dmochowski RR, et al. Best practice policy statement on urologic surgery antimicrobial prophylaxis. J Urol. 2008;180(5):2262–3.

7. Zani EL, Clark OA, Rodrigues NN. Antibiotic prophylaxis for transrectal prostate biopsy. Cochrane Database Syst Rev. 2011;5, CD006576.

8. Taylor AK, Zembower TR, Nadler RB, et al. Targeted antimicrobial prophylaxis using rectal swab cultures in men undergoing transrectal ultrasound guided prostate biopsy is associated with reduced incidence of postoperative infectious complications and cost of care. J Urol. 2012;187(4):1275–9.

9. Davis M, Sofer M, Kim SS, et al. The procedure of transrectal ultrasound guided biopsy of the prostate: a survey of patient preparation and biopsy technique. J Urol. 2002;167(2):566–70.

10. Carey JM, Korman HJ. Transrectal ultrasound guided biopsy of the prostate. Do enemas decrease clinically significant complications? J Urol. 2001;166(1):82–5.

11. Zaytoun OM, Thomas A, Moussa AS, et al. Morbidity of prostate biopsy following simplified versus complex preparation protocols: assessment of the risk factors. Urology. 2011;77(4):910–4.

12. Bruyère F, Faivre d'Arcier B, Haringanji DC, et al. Effect of patient position on pain experienced during prostate biopsy. Urol Int. 2007;78(4):351–5.

13. Issa MM, Bux S, Chung T, et al. A randomized prospective trial of intrarectal lidocaine for pain control during transrectal prostate biopsy: the Emory University experience. J Urol. 2000;164(2):397–9.

14. Autorino R, De Sio M, Di Lorzeno G, et al. How to decrease pain during transrectal ultrasound guided prostate biopsy: a look at the literature. J Urol. 2005;174(6):2091–7.

15. Richman JM, Carter HB, Hanna MH, et al. Efficacy of periprostatic local anesthetic for prostate biopsy analgesia: a meta-analysis. Urology. 2006;67(6):1224–8.

16. Rabets JC, Jones JS, Patel AR, et al. Bupivacaine provides rapid, effective periprostatic anaesthesia for transrectal prostate biopsy. BJU Int. 2004;93(9): 1216–7.

17. Lee-Elliott CE, Dundas D, Patel U. Randomized trial of lidocaine vs lidocaine/bupivacaine periprostatic injection on longitudinal pain scores after prostate biopsy. J Urol. 2004;171:247–50.

18. Rodriguez A, Kyriakou G, Leray E, et al. Prospective study comparing two methods of anaesthesia for prostate biopsies: apex periprostatic nerve block versus intrarectal lidocaine gel: review of the literature. Eur Urol. 2003;44(2):195–200.

19. Giannarini G, Autorino R, Valent F, et al. Combination of perianal-intrarectal lidocaine-prilocaine cream and periprostatic nerve block for pain control during transrectal ultrasound guided prostate biopsy: a randomized, controlled trial. J Urol. 2009;181(2):585–91.

20. Cantiello F, Cicione A, Autorino R, et al. Pelvic plexus block is more effective than periprostatic nerve block for pain control during office transrectal ultrasound guided prostate biopsy: a single center, prospective, randomized, double arm study. J Urol. 2012; 188(2):417–22.

21. Onur R, Littrup PJ, Pontes JE, et al. Contemporary impact of transrectal ultrasound lesions for prostate cancer detection. J Urol. 2004;172(2):512–4.

22. Spajic B, Eupic H, Tomas D, et al. The incidence of hyperechoic prostate cancer in transrectal ultrasound-guided biopsy specimens. Urology. 2007;70(4):734–7.

23. Patel AR, Jones JS. The prostate needle biopsy gun: busting a myth. J Urol. 2007;178(2):683–5.

24. Bratt O. The difficult case in prostate cancer diagnosis—when is a 'diagnostic TURP' indicated? Eur Urol. 2006; 49(5):769–71.

25. Hara R, Jo Y, Fujii T, et al. Optimal approach for prostate cancer detection as initial biopsy: prospective randomized study comparing transperineal versus transrectal systematic 12-core biopsy. Urology. 2008; 71(2):191–5.

26. Ching CB, Moussa AS, Li J, et al. Does transrectal ultrasound probe configuration relay matter? End fire versus side fire probe prostate cancer detection rates. J Urol. 2009;181(5):2077–82.

27. Ching CB, Zaytoun O, Moussa AS, et al. Type of transrectal ultrasonography probe influences prostate cancer detection rates on repeat prostate biopsy. BJU Int. 2012. doi:10.1111/j.1464-410X.2011.10689.x.

28. Rom M, Pycha A, Wiunig C, et al. Prospective randomized multicenter study comparing prostate cancer detection rates of end-fire and side-fire transrectal ultrasound probe configuration. Urology. 2012;80(1):15–8.

29. Eskew LA, Bare RL, McCullough DL. Systematic 5 region prostate biopsy is superior to sextant method for diagnosing carcinoma of the prostate. J Urol. 1997;157(1):199–202.

30. Presti JC, O'Dowd GJ, Miller MC, et al. Extended peripheral zone biopsy schemes increase cancer detection rates and minimize variance in prostate specific antigen and age related cancer rates: results of a community multi-practice study. J Urol. 2003;169:125–9.

31. Moussa AS, Meshref A, Schoenfield L, et al. Importance of additional "extreme" anterior apical needle biopsies in the initial detection of prostate cancer. Urology. 2010;75(5):1034–9.

32. Borboroglu PG, Comer SW, Riffenburgh RH, et al. Extensive repeat transrectal ultrasound guided prostate biopsy in patient with previous benign negative sextant biopsies. J Urol. 2000;163:158–62.

33. Jones JS, Oder M, Zippe CD. Saturation prostate biopsy with periprostatic block can be performed in office. J Urol. 2002;168(5):2108–10.

34. Jones JS, Patel A, Schoenfield L, et al. Saturation technique does not improve cancer detection as an initial prostate biopsy strategy. J Urol. 2006;175(2):485–8.

35. Jones JS, Zippe CD. Rectal sensation test helps avoid pain of apical prostate biopsy. J Urol. 2003;170: 2316–8.
36. Rodriguez LV, Terris MK. Risks and complications of transrectal ultrasound guided prostate needle biopsy: a prospective study and review of the literature. J Urol. 1998;160:2115–20.
37. Raajimakers R, Kirkels WF, Roobol MJ, et al. Complication rates and risk factors of 5802 transrectal ultrasound-guided sextant biopsies of the prostate within a population-based screening program. Urology. 2002;60:826–30.
38. Ecke TH, Gunia S, Bartel P, et al. Complications and risk factors of transrectal ultrasound guided needle biopsies of the prostate evaluated by questionnaire. Urol Oncol. 2008;26(5):474–8.
39. Pinkhasov GI, Lin YK, Palmerola R, et al. Complications following prostate needle biopsy requiring hospital admission or emergency department visits—experience from 1000 consecutive cases. BJU Int. 2012;110(3):369–74.
40. Liss MA, Change A, Santos R, et al. Prevalence and significant of fluoroquinolone resistant Escherichia coli in patients undergoing transrectal ultrasound guided prostate needle biopsy. J Urol. 2011;185(4):1283–8.
41. Nak RK, Saskin R, Lee Y, et al. Increasing hospital admission rates for urological complications after transrectal ultrasound guided prostate biopsy. J Urol. 2010;183:963–8.
42. Klein T, Palisaar RJ, Holz A, et al. The impact of prostate biopsy and periprostatic nerve block on erectile and voiding dysfunction: a prospective study. J Urol. 2010;184(4):1447–52.
43. Fujita K, Landis P, McNeil BK, et al. Serial prostate biopsy are associated with an increased risk of erectile dysfunction in men with prostate cancer and active surveillance. J Urol. 2009;182(6):2664–9.
44. Maccagnano C, Gallina A, Roscigno M, et al. Prostate saturation biopsy following a first negative biopsy: state of the art. Urol Int. 2012;89(2):126–35.
45. Zaytoun OM, Moussa AM, Gao T, et al. Office based transrectal saturation biopsy improves prostate cancer detection compared to extended biopsy in the repeat biopsy population. J Urol. 2011;186(3):850–4.
46. Patel AR, Jones JS, Rabets J, et al. Parasagittal biopsies add minimal information in repeat saturation prostate biopsy. Urology. 2004;63:87–9.
47. Djavan B, Ravery V, Zlotta A, et al. Prospective evaluation of prostate cancer detected on biopsies 1, 2, 3 and 4: when should we stop? J Urol. 2001;166: 1679–83.
48. Tan N, Lane BR, Li J, Moussa AS, Soriano M, Jones JS. Prostate cancers diagnosed at repeat biopsy are smaller and less likely to be high grade. J Urol. 2008; 180(4):1325–9.
49. Zaytoun OM, Stephenson AJ, Fareed K, et al. When serial prostate biopsy is recommended: most cancers detected are clinically insignificant. BJU Int. 2012. doi:10.1111/j.1464-410X.2012.10958.x.
50. Stoianovici D. Technology advances for prostate biopsy and needle therapies. J Urol. 2012. doi:10.1016/j.juro.2012.07.127.

Magnetic Resonance Imaging in Prostate Cancer Diagnosis

Srinivas Vourganti and Andrij R. Wojtowycz

Introduction

In recent years, prostate cancer-specific death rates have fallen significantly in industrialized nations, contributed in part by the widespread application of curative intent treatment and early disease detection afforded by PSA screening [1]. Unfortunately, this progress has been accompanied by the overtreatment of many patients likely to have never died of their prostate cancer. Distinguishing between clinically significant and indolent cancers is a major focus of current inquiry. Contemporary clinical screening regimens utilizing serum PSA and systematic transrectal ultrasound-guided biopsy suffer from poor sensitivity and specificity [2, 3] and ultimately lead to both overdetection of low-risk indolent disease as well as missed cancers of more clinical significance. This clinical uncertainty is reflected in the high upgrading rate of approximately 30 % between clinical diagnosis and radical prostatectomy [4]. As a result, neither clinician nor patient can rely on

clinical staging information with certainty in order to predict behavior. As a result, many men turn to more invasive and radical treatments even in the setting of predicted low-risk cancer, which while effective in controlling oncologic risk are associated with significant morbidity and cost.

Much investigative work has been performed in the hopes to improve and possibly remove this uncertainty. Recent advances in prostate cancer imaging, specifically those protocols which utilize 3 T Magnetic Resonance Imaging (MRI) coupled with an endorectal coil, have significantly improved the signal to noise ratio of image acquisition. As a result, a revolutionary improvement in temporal and spatial resolution has been achieved [5]. This imaging clarity has finally offered adequate insight into the three-dimensional anatomy of the gland to allow identification and characterization of individual prostate tumor lesions within the gland.

Moreover, by combining conventional anatomic MR imaging with advanced functional MR sequences (known as multiparametric imaging, including diffusion-weighted imaging, dynamic contrast-enhanced imaging, and spectroscopy), additional biophysical information can be gathered which allows true radiologic discernment between individual prostate cancer lesions and adjacent benign areas of the prostate [6, 7]. Initial reports at centers utilizing MRI in guiding diagnostic biopsy have shown it to be superior to established techniques of random sampling in the clinical diagnosis of disease [8, 9]. In this chapter, we aim to provide an overview of mpMRI of the prostate.

S. Vourganti, M.D. (✉)
Department of Urology, Urologic Oncology, State University of New York, Upstate Medical University, 750 East Adams Street, Syracuse, NY 13210, USA
e-mail: vourgans@upstate.edu

A.R. Wojtowycz, M.D.
Diagnostic Division, Department of Radiology, SUNY Upstate Medical University, Syracuse, NY, USA

R.V. Khanna et al. (eds.), *Surgical Techniques for Prostate Cancer*,
DOI 10.1007/978-1-4939-1616-0_3, © Springer Science+Business Media New York 2015

Multiparametric Magnetic Resonance Imaging

Multiparametric Magnetic Resonance Imaging (MP-MRI) is a noninvasive imaging technique with superior diagnostic characteristics in comparison to other imaging modalities such as ultrasound and computed tomography. Recent technologic advancements including high field strength magnets (3 T and greater) and new magnetic coil designs (including endorectal coil and multichannel surface coils) as well as advancements in software and computational algorithms have allowed the addition of more complex functional imaging to clinical imaging. Here we describe the four component parameters of a contemporary mp-MRI study.

T2-Weighted MRI (Anatomic Imaging)

T2-weighted anatomic imaging is the most commonly used and widely available imaging sequence. This modality provides excellent delineation of prostate zonal anatomy, gland borders, and visualization of surrounding tissues (Fig 3.1) [6]. Normal prostatic tissue exhibits relative high T2 signal intensity in the prostate peripheral zone (the origin of most adenocarcinoma lesions), and lower signal intensity in the central gland. Classically, prostate cancer lesions are noted to exhibit low signal intensity, a characteristic most easily visualized in the peripheral zone due to its normally higher signal intensity. Thus, rare transitional zone and central gland lesions are much more difficult to identify in this sequence. In addition, many benign conditions can mimic

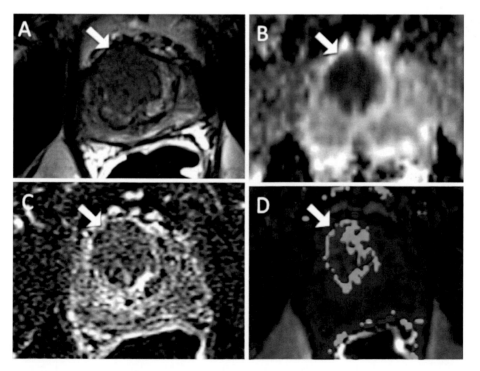

Fig. 3.1 Axial MRI images of the prostate: (**a**) Axial T2-weighted image of the prostate shows a large decreased signal intensity lesion in the right anterior mid-transitional zone (*arrow*). (**b**) DWI ADC map of the prostate shows restricted diffusion within this lesion (*arrow*).

(**c**) DCE-MRI subtracted contrast image clearly outlines the lesion (*arrow*). (**d**) DCE-MRI color map overlay indicates that the lesion is hypervascular with rapid contrast wash-in and wash-out (*arrow*)

this appearance of low signal intensity (such as inflammation). As a result, when relying on only this parameter approximately half of lesions are missed [10]. Also, not surprisingly, lesion size has significant impact on detection, with larger tumors (1 cm) nearly always visualized and smaller tumors (<5 mm) much more likely missed [11].

Owing to the detail of T2 imaging, it is the most helpful sequence for assessing local invasion into surrounding tissues. Detection of this local invasion has clinical relevance as it decreases the likelihood of cure from local therapy. Such invasion can be seen most overtly as direct invasion into the periprostatic fat. In addition, other findings suggestive of local invasion are irregularity of the gland margin, capsular bulge, and a low signal area within the seminal vesicles (which normally exhibit very high signal intensity). The results from such local staging predictions are not perfect, however, and absence of findings may occur in the setting of true disease with reports ranging with diagnostic sensitivity of 50–60 % [12, 13].

Diffusion-Weighted MRI

Diffusion-Weighted MRI (DW-MRI) sequences can detect and quantify the Brownian motion of water within tissue in vivo [14]. As this relates to cellular density, cell permeability, and free water diffusion within the interstitial spaces, DW-MRI can assess tissue structural architecture and differentiate benign tissue from malignant tissue. Benign tissue exhibits high signal intensity as it normally allows free water to diffuse with relative ease. In the malignant setting, relative higher nuclear:cytoplasmic ratio and loss of extracellular spaces due to cellular proliferation results in decreased free water diffusion and thus relative decreased signal intensity on DW-MRI [15]. Furthermore, DW-MRI findings have been significantly correlated to underlying histopathologic grade and clinical risk scores [16], which allows some prediction of tumor histopathologic behavior based on radiologic findings.

Downsides of DW-MRI include its relatively poor spatial resolution (especially in comparison to T2-weighted MRI) which limits the ability to evaluate staging using this sequence in isolation. In addition, DW-MRI is more challenging to interpret in the central gland as the presence of BPH-associated nodules in this area of the prostate can mimic the low signal intensity of malignant lesions [17]. Despite this, addition of DW-MRI to standard anatomic T2-weighted imaging has been demonstrated to improved diagnostic accuracy [10].

Dynamic Contrast-Enhanced Magnetic Resonance Imaging

Dynamic Contrast-Enhanced Magnetic Resonance Imaging (DCE-MRI) allows assessment of tissue vascular supply. This is accomplished by acquiring T1-weighted images continuously before, throughout, and continuing after the injection of an MRI detectable contrast agent (i.e., gadolinium). Signal increase during this protocol results from blood supply to the tissue of interest. Differentiation between normal and malignant tissue is possible, as cancers have a typical imaging signature owing to their disordered angiogenesis. Malignant tissue is correlated with early uptake and early washout (temporal imaging) of vascular contrast [18]. These changes are most easily seen in larger lesions and in lesions which are of higher grade. In addition, similar to T2-weighted and DWI-MRI, lesions in the central gland are more challenging to differentiate as BPH nodules themselves can show early uptake, though they do not classically have the rapid washout typical of malignant lesions. DCE-MRI has been shown to have higher diagnostic power than T2W sequences alone, especially in lesions larger than 5 mm [19]. Similar to DWI, DCE-MRI sequences have relatively poor spatial resolution (in comparison to T2-weighted MRI) which limits the ability to evaluate staging using this sequence in isolation. However, it is felt to be most useful in assessment treatment effect in settings where the prostate gland remains in situ.

Magnetic Resonance Spectroscopic Imaging

Nuclear magnetic resonance spectroscopy is possible in situ using Magnetic Resonance Spectroscopic Imaging (MRSI) which allows relative quantification of metabolites within the tissue of interest. In this technique, the tissue of interest is divided into discrete areas (volumes of interest) known as voxels. For each voxel, a spectra of EM radiation is acquired which represents a fingerprint of the composition of the volume. This data can be used to differentiate benign from malignant tissue. Benign prostate typically harbors high levels of citrate, which can be detected as a specific peak on MRSI spectra. In the setting of cancer, the increased cellular turnover results in a relatively high concentration of choline, also detectable on the MRSI spectral curve. From this data, the relative concentration of choline:citrate can be calculated, with increased ratios signifying malignant changes. The addition of MRSI has been shown to improve diagnostic accuracy over T2-weighted imaging alone, with especially high specificity [20]. Some challenges to this technique are that inflammation can mimic citrate:choline signal changes, and that spatial resolution (similar to DWI and DCE-MRI) is not as good as T2-weighted MRI in the aid of local staging. In addition, some centers report that it is technically challenging and on some platforms it increases acquisition times limiting its widespread utilization.

MP-MRI: Combining Imaging Parameters for Improved Diagnostic Power

As each individual parameter is capturing orthogonal data, the combination of them has been demonstrated to have improved diagnostic power over each individual in isolation. Using careful histopathologic correlation of radical prostatectomy specimens, it has been demonstrated that a lesion identified has a positive predictive value of 98 %, with excellent sensitivity especially in larger lesions of clinical significance (>5 mm) [20].

Harnessing the Diagnostic Power of MRI: MRI Targeted Biopsy

A number of strategies have been employed to take advantage of this additional diagnostic information from MRI. While in gantry biopsy has been performed to directly sample areas of suspicion, the added imaging time and need for specialized non-ferrous equipment makes it difficult to implement widely and in a cost-effective manner. Most contemporary strategies target areas of suspicion in an outpatient setting following a priori evaluation of MRI imaging by an experienced radiologist. The most popular methods employ software-based co-registration systems, known as fusion MRI-US biopsy (Fig 3.2). These systems utilize mechanically encoded biopsy arms or electromagnetic tracking to guide the needle to aforementioned areas of suspicion using software calculations which correlate MRI findings with real-time US data. Preliminary reports demonstrate excellent diagnostic power utilizing these strategies with improved sensitivity, specificity, and decreased upgrading rate [21]. In addition, manual targeting has been performed (so called "cognitive" biopsy), and in experienced hands, has been able to approximate the improved diagnostic power of computer-aided fusion-based systems [22].

While data is still preliminary, early results of the performance of MR imaging have been promising. Such strategies have proved useful in challenging situations such as persistent clinical suspicion in the setting of prior negative biopsy [9], as well as more accurately characterizing appropriate candidates considering active surveillance [23].

Conclusion

MRI of the prostate has offered additional diagnostic certainty in the setting of prostate cancer diagnosis over established standard of care methods. Contemporary experience is still very preliminary; however, it is likely that MRI will be utilized in all stages of prostate cancer diagnostics including staging, guiding of therapy, and follow-up after treatment.

Fig. 3.2 Real-time transrectal ultrasound image (*top panel*) co-registered with MRI reconstruction data (*bottom panel*) using MRI-US Fusion software. This allows needle targeting of a predetermined area of suspicion (*blue* and *red* target) which is dynamically overlayed onto both images simultaneously

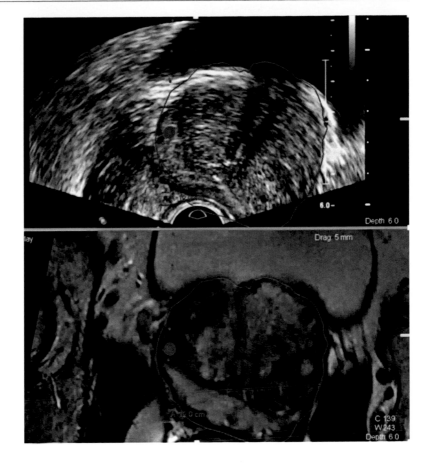

References

1. Jemal A, et al. Global cancer statistics. CA Cancer J Clin. 2011;61(2):69–90.
2. Ouzaid I, et al. A direct comparison of the diagnostic accuracy of three prostate cancer nomograms designed to predict the likelihood of a positive initial transrectal biopsy. Prostate. 2012;72:1200–6.
3. Haas GP, et al. Needle biopsies on autopsy prostates: sensitivity of cancer detection based on true prevalence. J Natl Cancer Inst. 2007;99(19):1484–9.
4. Tilki D, et al. Clinical and pathologic predictors of Gleason sum upgrading in patients after radical prostatectomy: results from a single institution series. Urol Oncol. 2011;29(5):508–14.
5. Lagemaat MW, Scheenen TW. Role of high-field MR in studies of localized prostate cancer. NMR Biomed. 2014;27(1):67–79.
6. Turkbey B, et al. Prostate cancer: value of multiparametric MR imaging at 3 T for detection-histopathologic correlation. Radiology. 2010;255(1):89–99.
7. Panebianco V, et al. Conventional imaging and multiparametric magnetic resonance (MRI, MRS, DWI, MRP) in the diagnosis of prostate cancer. Q J Nucl Med Mol Imaging. 2012;56(4):331–42.
8. Pinto PA, et al. Magnetic resonance imaging/ultrasound fusion guided prostate biopsy improves cancer detection following transrectal ultrasound biopsy and correlates with multiparametric magnetic resonance imaging. J Urol. 2011;186(4):1281–5.
9. Vourganti S, et al. Multiparametric magnetic resonance imaging and ultrasound fusion biopsy detect prostate cancer in patients with prior negative transrectal ultrasound biopsies. J Urol. 2012;188(6):2152–7.
10. Haider MA, et al. Combined T2-weighted and diffusion-weighted MRI for localization of prostate cancer. AJR Am J Roentgenol. 2007;189(2):323–8.
11. Nakashima J, et al. Endorectal MRI for prediction of tumor site, tumor size, and local extension of prostate cancer. Urology. 2004;64(1):101–5.
12. Park BK, et al. Comparison of phased-array 3.0-T and endorectal 1.5-T magnetic resonance imaging in the evaluation of local staging accuracy for prostate cancer. J Comput Assist Tomogr. 2007;31:534–8.
13. Futterer JJ, et al. Staging prostate cancer with dynamic contrast-enhanced endorectal MR imaging prior to radical prostatectomy: experienced versus less experienced readers. Radiology. 2005;237:541–9.
14. Issa B, et al. In vivo measurement of the apparent diffusion coefficient in normal and malignant prostatic

tissues using echo-planar imaging. J Magn Reson Imaging. 2002;16(2):196.

15. Lim KS, et al. Diffusion weighted MRI of adult male pelvic cancers. Clin Radiol. 2012;67:899.

16. Turkbey B, et al. Is apparent diffusion coefficient associated with clinical risk scores for prostate cancers that are visible on 3-T MR images? Radiology. 2011;258(2):488–95.

17. Oto A, et al. Prostate cancer: differentiation of central gland cancer from benign prostatic hyperplasia by using diffusion weighted and dynamic contrast enhanced MR imaging. Radiology. 2010; 257:715.

18. Verma S, et al. Overview of dynamic contrast-enhanced MRI in prostate cancer diagnosis and management. AJR Am J Roentgenol. 2012;198(6): 1277–88.

19. Puech P, et al. Dynamic contrast-enhanced-magnetic resonance imaging evaluation of intraprostatic prostate

cancer: correlation with radical prostatectomy specimens. Urology. 2009;74(5):1094–9.

20. Turkbey B, et al. Multiparametric 3 T prostate magnetic resonance imaging to detect cancer: histopathological correlation using prostatectomy specimens processed in customized magnetic resonance imaging based molds. J Urol. 2011;186(5):1818–24.

21. Le JD et al. MRI-ultrasound fusion biopsy for prediction of final prostate pathology. J Urol. 2014;pii: S0022-5347(14)03509-5

22. Wysock JS et al. A prospective, blinded comparison of magnetic resonance (MR) imaging-ultrasound fusion and visual estimation in the performance of MR-targeted prostate biopsy: The PROFUS Trial. Eur Urol. 2013;pii:S0302-2838(13)01186-X

23. Stamatakis L, et al. Accuracy of multiparametric magnetic resonance imaging in confirming eligibility for active surveillance for men with prostate cancer. Cancer. 2013;119(18):3359–66.

Open Radical Retropubic Prostatectomy and Pelvic Lymph Node Dissection

4

Joseph C. Klink and Eric A. Klein

Preoperative Preparation

All patients meet with the surgical team (surgeon and midlevel provider), preferably including partners, for discussion of the general nature of the procedure, potential complications-anticipated course and recovery of continence and potency, and the postoperative routine. Specific emphasis is placed on the use of epidural anesthesia, whether or not lymphadenectomy is to be performed, whether or not a nerve sparing procedure is contemplated, planned hospital length of stay (typically 24 h), and time to return to normal activity (typically 2 and half weeks). A preoperative urinalysis should demonstrate no active infection. No preoperative dietary restrictions and no bowel preparation are used. Patients are admitted to the operating room (OR) on the day of surgery. A second-generation cephalosporin, or vancomycin and gentamycin if allergic to penicillin or cepahalosporins, is given intravenously just prior to incision and for two doses postoperatively.

J.C. Klink, M.D. (✉)
Glickman Urological and Kidney Institute, Center
for Urologic Oncology, Cleveland Clinic Foundation,
Cleveland, OH, USA
e-mail: klinkj@ccf.org

E.A. Klein, M.D.
Glickman Urological and Kidney Institute,
Cleveland Clinic Foundation, Cleveland, OH, USA

Intermittent compression stockings are used for prophylaxis against deep venous thrombosis. Subcutaneous heparin is not used.

Anesthetic Considerations

Epidural anesthesia alone is the preferred technique for all patients. The epidural catheter is placed in low thoracic position preoperatively and dosed with 0.1 % bupivacaine and morphine sulfate 0.05 mg/mL upon arrival in the OR. This combination of position and drugs has been demonstrated to promote early return of intestinal function by sympathetic blockade and results in less postoperative pain by induction of preemptive analgesia [1]. Analgesia is maintained intra- and postoperatively with morphine sulfate or fentanyl, and low doses of anxiolytics are given parenterally throughout the procedure as needed. Epidural anesthesia avoids the need for ventilatory support and eliminates pulmonary and laryngeal complications, causes less sedation, results in less narcotic use, requires fewer transfusions, and is less expensive than general anesthesia [2].

Patient Positioning

The patient is placed in the supine position with the table in mild reverse Trendelenburg position to facilitate exposure of the apex. Once the apical dissection is completed, the table is placed in mild

R.V. Khanna et al. (eds.), *Surgical Techniques for Prostate Cancer*,
DOI 10.1007/978-1-4939-1616-0_4, © Springer Science+Business Media New York 2015

Trendelenburg position to facilitate visualization and dissection of the bladder neck. Hyperextension of the table is not used as the exposure of the apex is usually adequate with reverse Trendelenburg alone. This also avoids nerve and soft tissue injury that may result from hyperextension of the spine for a prolonged period.

Incision, Exposure, and Retractor Placement

An 18-French Foley catheter is placed transurethrally, and the balloon is inflated with 10 cm³ of water prior to incision. A midline incision is made from below the umbilicus to the top of the pubis (Fig. 4.1), typically 8 cm in length. The space of Retzius is developed bluntly, and the bladder is mobilized off the pelvic sidewall bilaterally. The peritoneum is also mobilized superiorly, exposing the psoas muscles bilaterally. The vas deferens is not routinely divided. A Bookwalter retractor with blades specifically

modified for the performance of radical prostatectomy is placed (Fig. 4.2) [3]. Two body wall retractor blades on both sides of the incision are usually adequate. A midline suprapubic blade is not routinely used. When pelvic lymphadenectomy is performed, a malleable blade is secured to the ring for lateral retraction of the bladder, permitting full visualization of the obturator fossa (Fig. 4.3).

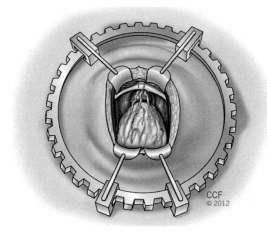

Fig. 4.2 A self-retaining, table-fixed ring retractor is placed. The prostatic apex is to the top. Reprinted with permission, Cleveland Clinic Center for Medical Art & Photography © 1996–2013. All Rights Reserved

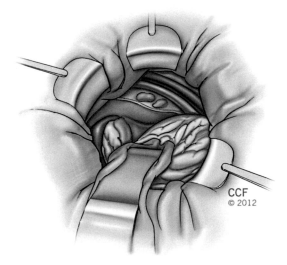

Fig. 4.3 A malleable blade is used for exposure of the obturator fossa when pelvic lymphadenectomy is performed. Reprinted with permission, Cleveland Clinic Center for Medical Art & Photography © 1996–2013. All Rights Reserved

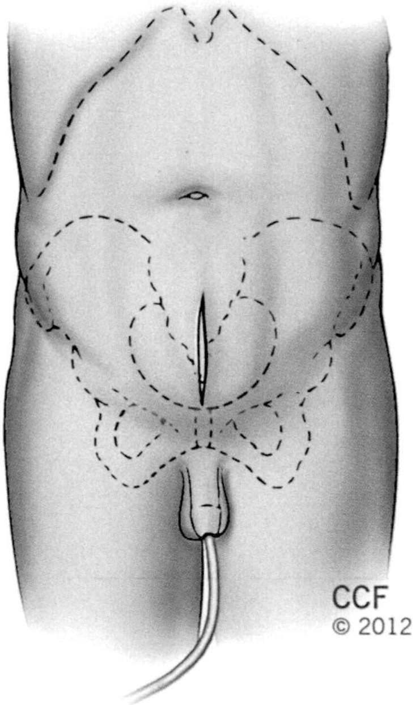

Fig. 4.1 An 18-French Foley catheter is placed transurethrally, and an extraperitoneal incision is made in the lower midline, approximately 8 cm in length. Reprinted with permission, Cleveland Clinic Center for Medical Art & Photography © 1996–2013. All Rights Reserved

Pelvic Lymphadenectomy

Based on published nomograms and our own experience, pelvic lymphadenectomy is omitted in selected patients at low risk for lymph node metastases based on preoperative serum prostate-specific antigen (PSA), tumor grade, and palpable tumor extent. Generally, lymphadenectomy is omitted in patients with AUA or D'Amico low-risk criteria. Such patients have a minuscule risk of positive nodes and omission of lymphadenectomy in patients with these characteristics does not increase the likelihood of biochemical failure [4]. For prognostic and potential therapeutic purposes, an extended lymphadenectomy is performed in all patients not meeting the low risk criteria. The dissection includes the tissue medial to the external iliac artery, all tissue surrounding the external iliac, the internal iliac artery superiorally, the bifurcation of the external and internal iliac veins cephalad, the origin of the superficial circumflex iliac vein caudally, and the pelvic sidewall in the obturator fossa deeply. In addition, the nodes immediately medial to the common iliac artery are excised. The extent of the dissection is guided by the study by Mattei et al. showing that the nodes within these boundaries constitute 75 % of the primary lymphatic drainage of the prostate [5]. Frozen section analysis is not routinely performed unless the nodes are grossly suspicious, and only if a finding of positive nodes would result in aborting the prostatectomy.

Endopelvic and Lateral Pelvic Fascia, Santorini's Plexus, and Dorsal Vein Complex

The apical dissection begins with vertical incisions of the endopelvic fascia at the apex bilaterally (Fig. 4.4). The attachments of the levator muscles to the lateral surface of the prostate are taken down sharply with scissors. Blunt dissection of these attachments should be avoided to prevent shearing of small blood vessels, which may be difficult to control. The puboprostatic ligaments are divided.

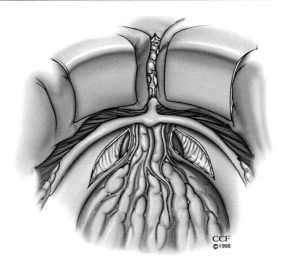

Fig. 4.4 The endopelvic fascia is incised bilaterally just lateral to the prostatic apex. The attachments of the levator muscles to the lateral surface of the prostate are taken down sharply with scissors. The puboprostatic ligaments are left intact. The apex is to the top. Reprinted with permission, Cleveland Clinic Center for Medical Art & Photography © 1996–2013. All Rights Reserved

Next, the lateral pelvic fascia (the visceral portion of the endopelvic fascia) covering the prostate is incised bilaterally beginning from the initial incision in the apical endopelvic fascia and extending to the base of the prostate (Fig. 4.5). The incision is performed high on the lateral surface of the prostate to avoid injuring the neurovascular bundles (NVBs). When completed, this maneuver allows clear visualization of the prostatourethral junction and location of the NVBs and facilitates bunching of the ramifications of the dorsal vein over the prostate. The cut edges of the lateral fascia are then grasped with Turner-Babcock clamps, incorporating the branches of the venous plexus on the dorsolateral surface of the prostate (Fig. 4.6a). The bunched tissue is suture-ligated with two individual figure-of-8 0-chromic ligatures (Fig. 4.6b, c). This technique is a modification of the dorsal venous plexus bunching technique originally described by Myers [6]. It prevents back-bleeding when the dorsal vein is divided and helps identify the plane between the dorsal vein and urethra. The prostate is next retracted superiorly with a sponge stick, and the fat between the puboprostatic ligaments

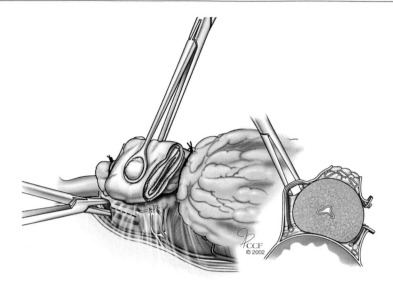

Fig. 4.5 The lateral pelvic fascia (the visceral layer of the endopelvic fascia covering the prostate) is elevated with a right-angled clamp and incised sharply with a knife (along the *dotted line*) from the apex to base of the prostate. This maneuver exposes the anterior prostatourethral junction and the position of the neurovascular bundles and facilitates control of the ramifications of the dorsal vein over the prostate. The maneuver is then repeated on the opposite side (not shown). The apex is to the left. Reprinted with permission, Cleveland Clinic Center for Medical Art & Photography © 1996–2013. All Rights Reserved

is gently removed to expose the superficial dorsal vein which is then divided between clips.

The dorsal vein and urethra are closely approximated and passage of an instrument between them carries the risk of damaging the anterior-striated sphincter. Therefore, the dorsal vein is next divided with scissors, exposing the anterior surface of the urethra (Fig. 4.7a). The distal portion of the incised dorsal vein is then oversewn with a figure-of-8 suture using a 3-0 absorbable monofilament suture on a 26 mm 5/8 circle needle (Fig. 4.7b). When correctly performed this technique does not compromise the anterior prostatic margin and results in excellent visualization of the urethra (Fig. 4.7c).

Release of NVBs

For nerve-sparing procedures, the NVBs are next released from the prostate from the apex to the level of the vascular pedicle lateral to the seminal vesicles. The dissection is performed with tenotomy scissors and begins at the mid-prostate with identification of the most superior peri-prostatic vein, which marks the upper extent of the bundle. The dissection is carried sharply around the edge of the prostate bilaterally, entering the plane posterior to Denonvilliers' fascia and anterior to the rectum (Fig. 4.8). This plane is fully developed by sharp dissection, using a sponge stick for gentle rotation of the prostate (Fig. 4.8a); blunt dissection with an instrument or finger runs the risk of fracturing the neurovascular bundle and should be avoided. When this plane is fully developed, the prostate can be lifted off the rectal surface (Fig. 4.8b). This maneuver yields excellent visualization of the prostatourethral junction both anteriorly and posteriorly and allows precise transection of the urethra without risk of incision into the prostatic apex. For a non-nerve-sparing procedure, the incision in the lateral pelvic fascia is made lateral to the bundles to permit wide excision of all periprostatic tissue (Fig. 4.8c). The plane between the prostate and rectum is developed similarly.

There are several advantages to the described approach. Initial release of the lateral pelvic fascia allows superior visualization of the junction

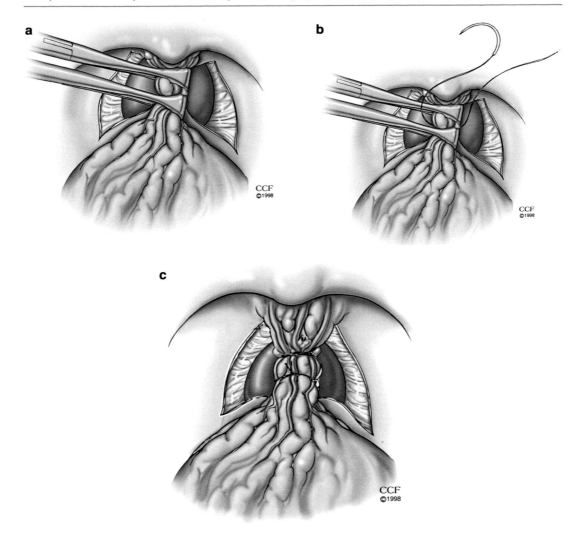

Fig. 4.6 Bunching technique for control of the dorsal venous complex. (**a**) Turner-Babcock clamps are used to bunch together the branches of the dorsal vein covering the dorsal surface of the prostate. (**b**) Two figure-of-8 sutures are used to ligate these branches, incorporating the cut edges of the endopelvic fascia. (**c**) Appearance after both sutures have been placed. The apex is to the top. Reprinted with permission, Cleveland Clinic Center for Medical Art & Photography © 1996–2013. All Rights Reserved

between the rectum and prostate, with precise definition of the plane of dissection between these organs leaving all layers of Denonvilliers' fascia on the prostate. This reduces the likelihood of a positive margin along the posterior aspect of this fascia. Lifting the prostate off the rectum early in the dissection also permits precise delineation of the anatomy of the prostatic apex, especially posterior to the urethra, and prevents leaving small amounts of prostatic tissue attached to the urethra.

Improved visualization of the apex using this technique also incorporates one of the main advantages of the perineal approach while still permitting adequate visualization and resection of the bladder neck and seminal vesicles. This technique also fully preserves the posterior fascial attachments of the urethra. Finally, dissection of the neurovascular bundles away from the prostate prior to transection of the urethra lowers the risk of traction injury when the apex is elevated.

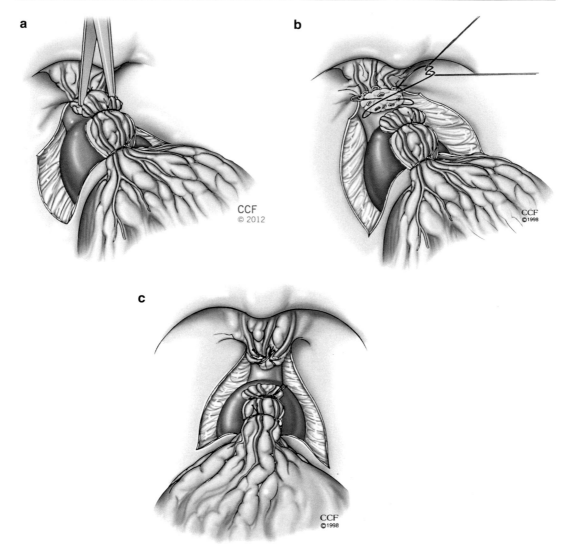

Fig. 4.7 Division and control of the dorsal vein. The prostatic apex is to the left. (**a**) The dorsal vein is divided with scissors, exposing the anterior surface of the urethra. (**b**) The cut surface of the dorsal vein is suture-ligated for hemostasis. (**c**) Appearance of the urethra after division and ligation of the dorsal vein. Reprinted with permission, Cleveland Clinic Center for Medical Art & Photography © 1996–2013. All Rights Reserved

Division of the Urethra and Placement of Urethrovesical Sutures

Following division of the dorsal vein complex and release of the lateral fascia and NVBs, the prostate remains attached at the apex only by the urethra. Division of the urethra begins with an incision of the anterior surface between 3- and 9-o'clock

(Fig. 4.9a), exposing the Foley catheter. The catheter is next removed to allow placement of the vesicourethral anastomotic sutures. Placement of these sutures is facilitated by leaving the posterior urethra attached to the prostate in order to prevent urethral retraction (Fig. 4.9b). Five sutures of absorbable material are used for the anastomosis, placed at the 12-, 3-, 5-, 7-, and 9-o'clock positions, taking care to avoid the NVBs lying posterolaterally. With experience placement of these

Fig. 4.8 Release of the neurovascular bundles. The prostatic apex is to the left. (**a**) The left neurovascular bundle is exposed by rotating the prostate medially with a sponge stick and released from the prostate by sharp dissection from the apex to the posterior vascular pedicle. The *inset* shows the plane of dissection medial to the bundle and posterior to Denonvilliers fascia. A similar dissection is performed on the other side. (**b**) The finger in the figure illustrates that when the dissection is complete, the prostate can be lifted off the anterior surface of the rectum. The dissection is not done bluntly with a finger. The urethra remains intact at this point of the dissection. (**c**) The dissection is similar for non-nerve-sparing procedures, except that the lateral fascia is incised lateral to the neurovascular bundles. The plane between the prostate and rectum is developed similarly to the nerve-sparing technique. Reprinted with permission, Cleveland Clinic Center for Medical Art & Photography © 1996–2013. All Rights Reserved

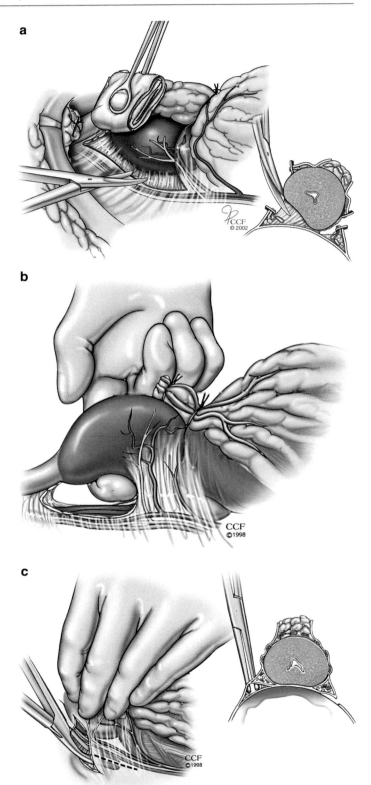

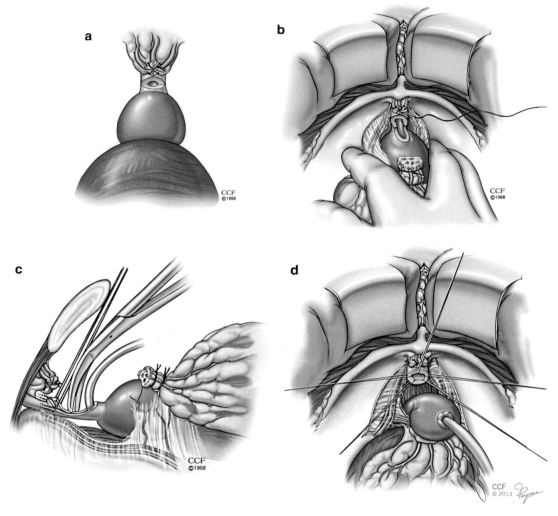

Fig. 4.9 Urethral division and placement of urethral sutures. (**a**) The anterior urethra is incised sharply from the 3- to 9-o'clock position, exposing the Foley catheter. (**b**) The Foley catheter is removed, and two anterior and three posterior anastomotic sutures are placed at the 12-, 3-, 5-, 7, and 9-o'clock positions, respectively. Leaving the posterior urethra attached facilitates suture placement by preventing urethral retraction. (**c**) The posterior urethra is divided sharply under direct vision, using gentle traction on the apex of the prostate for exposure. (**d**) Final appearance of the divided urethra with anastomotic sutures in place. Reprinted with permission, Cleveland Clinic Center for Medical Art & Photography © 1996–2013. All Rights Reserved

sutures can usually be easily accomplished from outside to inside without the need for double-armed sutures or a urethral sound. The sutures with needles still attached are held with hemostats labeled with the corresponding clock face position to avoid entanglement until the anastomosis is completed. Urethral transection, including the underlying layers of Denonvilliers' fascia, is next completed under direct vision using scissors and gentle traction on the prostatic apex for exposure (Fig. 4.9c, d). To minimize traction injury, the Foley catheter is not replaced into the prostate until the NVBs are fully released by division of the posterolateral pedicles.

Posterior Vascular Pedicles, Bladder Neck, and Seminal Vesicles

Dissection of the posterior vascular pedicles is easily accomplished after completion of the apical dissection. Placing the table in mild Trendelenburg position and gentle traction on the prostate facilitates visualization for this portion of the procedure. It has generally been our approach to perform the bladder neck dissection prior to dissection of the seminal vesicles to permit leaving as much fascia as possible on both sides of these glands, although the "posterior peel" technique of seminal vesicle dissection prior to bladder neck dissection is occasionally helpful for glands with large median lobes. Dissection of the prostate base begins with opening of the plane between the caudad surface of the seminal vesicles (still covered by Denonvillier's fascia) and the rectum to fully expose the medial surface of the posterior vascular pedicles. Lateral to the pedicles, the NVBs are typically tethered to the prostate by several 1 mm arterial branches, which are divided between small hemostatic clips to fully release them from the prostate.

The pedicles are similarly divided between clips, exposing the lateral surface of the seminal vesicles (Fig. 4.10). A small window is made sharply in Denonvillier's fascia over the seminal vesicle bilaterally, and the fascia and vessel-containing tissue lateral to the SVs is divided between clips. Next, a right-angled clamp is passed between the posterior bladder neck and cephalad surface of the seminal vesicles (Fig. 4.11a). The bladder neck is then incised sharply in a direction that preserves its anatomical integrity as much as possible and avoids cutting into the trigone near the ureteral orifices (Fig. 4.11b). In cases of high-grade or large volume tumor at the prostate base, a larger cuff of bladder neck is removed to ensure an adequate margin of normal tissue. Release of the prostate from the bladder neck exposes the posterior surface of the vas deferens and seminal vesicles (Fig. 4.11c). The vas are individually ligated with clips and divided; the remaining attachments of the seminal vesicles are then dissected sharply (Fig. 4.11d), ligating the small arterial branch at the tips of the glands, and the specimen is removed. In patients with low-risk disease, it is not necessary to excise the entirety of the seminal vesicles.

Fig. 4.10 The posterior vascular pedicles are divided bilaterally between clips. This exposes the junction of the bladder and prostate. Reprinted with permission, Cleveland Clinic Center for Medical Art & Photography © 1996–2013. All Rights Reserved

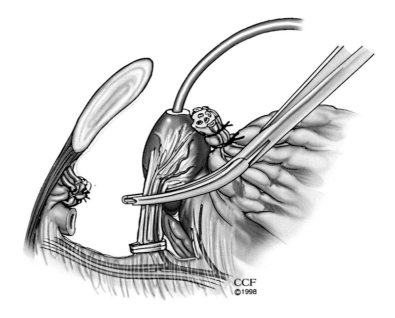

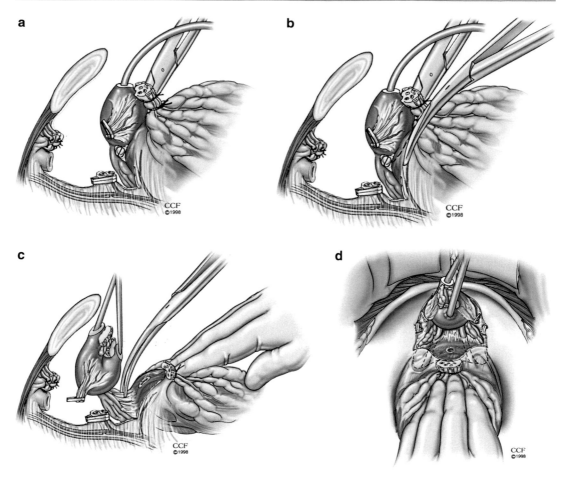

Fig. 4.11 Bladder neck dissection. (**a**) A right-angled clamp is inserted in the plane between the posterior bladder neck and the seminal vesicles. This maneuver helps identify the correct plane for bladder neck dissection without injury to the trigone. (**b**) The bladder neck is incised sharply, leaving an adequate cuff of bladder neck on the prostate while preserving the anatomical integrity of the bladder neck muscle fibers. (**c**) Release of the pros-tate from the bladder neck exposes the posterior surface of the vas deferens and seminal vesicles. The vasa are ligated with clips and divided. (**d**) The attachments to the seminal vesicles are divided, and the specimen is removed. Reprinted with permission, Cleveland Clinic Center for Medical Art & Photography © 1996–2013. All Rights Reserved

Completion of the Anastomosis

The final step is completion of the vesicourethral anastomosis. When necessary, the bladder neck is reconstructed using 3-0 chromic suture. The anastomotic sutures previously placed in the urethra are placed in corresponding positions in the bladder neck (Fig. 4.12a), placing the 5- and 7 o'clock sutures close to the midline to ensure a watertight closure posteriorly. A 20-French Foley catheter is then placed per urethra and guided into the bladder; the ballon is inflated with 10 cm³ of water. The cephalad two retractor blades (Fig. 4.2) are removed, releasing the bladder into the pelvis. The needles are removed from the sutures and the sutures are tied sequentially, beginning posteriorly (Fig. 4.12b). Use of a Foley with an overinflated balloon and traction on the bladder neck prior to tying the sutures is avoided, as the balloon simply fills up the already

Fig. 4.12 Vesicourethral anastomosis. (**a**) The five urethral sutures are placed into the bladder neck at the corresponding positions after eversion of the bladder neck mucosa. The *inset* shows detail of bladder neck suture placement after mucosal eversion. (**b**) The vesicourethral sutures are tied circumferentially over a 20-French Foley catheter (*left*). The final appearance of the completed anastomosis is illustrated (*right*). Reprinted with permission, Cleveland Clinic Center for Medical Art & Photography © 1996–2013. All Rights Reserved

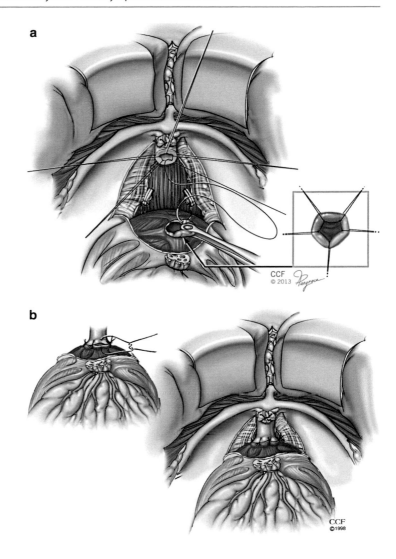

small space of the pelvis and may prevent good approximation of the bladder neck and urethra. An overinflated Foley balloon can also increase bladder spasms and obstruct the eye of the catheter. The anastomosis is checked for watertightness by irrigation via the Foley.

Closed suction drains are placed through separate incisions through the body of the rectus muscle and left in the obturator fossa. Only a single drain is used in patients in whom no pelvic lymphadenectomy is performed. The incision is closed in a single layer with running nonabsorbable suture, and the skin is approximated with clips.

Post-op Routine

Patients are ambulated and begin a clear liquid diet on the evening of surgery. Patient-controlled analgesia is maintained with continuous and on-demand morphine sulfate plus bupivacaine via epidural catheter for 24 h, followed by iv/po ketorolac and ibuprofen as needed. No oral or systemic narcotics are used. The drains are removed before discharge unless there is clinical suspicion of a urine leak. Approximately 90 % of patients are discharged to home on the first postoperative day. Patients return seven days after discharge for incisional staple and catheter removal. Cystograms are not routinely performed. In cases where the vesicourethral anastomosis is not tension-free and in cases of documented urine leak, the Foley is left in longer and a cystogram may be performed before catheter removal.

References

1. Scheinin B, Asantila R, Orko R. The effect of bupivacaine and morphine on pain and bowel function after colonic surgery. Acta Anaesthesiol Scand. 1987;31(2): 161–4.

2. Klein E. Contemporary technique of radical prostatectomy. In: Klein E, editor. Management of prostate cancer. Totowa, NJ: Humana; 2004. pp. 217–42.

3. Klein E. Modification of the Bookwalter retractor for radical prostatectomy. Contemp Urol. 1998;10: 65–9.

4. Weight CJ, et al. Limited pelvic lymph node dissection does not improve biochemical relapse-free survival at 10 years after radical prostatectomy in patients with low-risk prostate cancer. Urology. 2008;71(1):141–5.

5. Mattei A, et al. The template of the primary lymphatic landing sites of the prostate should be revisited: results of a multimodality mapping study. Eur Urol. 2008;53(1):118–25.

6. Myers RP. Improving the exposure of the prostate in radical retropubic prostatectomy: longitudinal bunching of the deep venous plexus. J Urol. 1989;142(5): 1282–4.

Laparoscopic Prostatectomy and Pelvic Lymph Node Dissection

5

Itay Sternberg, Guilherme Maia, Abdelkarim Touijer, and Bertrand D. Guillonneau

Fifteen years after the wide introduction of laparoscopy for prostate cancer surgery, there are little debates about the objective advantages of this approach over the open retropubic surgery, but there is still a debate about the best way to teach surgeons who want to dedicate themselves to minimally approaches for radical prostatectomy, this procedure being still one of the most complex procedures in urology at large, and specifically in uro-oncology.

Difficult first because the indications for radical prostatectomy are moving and fuzzy, what was the rule yesterday is in question today, and all these questions will not be answered before a long while. This uncertainty places the uro-oncologist in a peculiar position when he/she sets the indication for radical prostatectomy and engages his/her responsibility.

Responsibility in the indication: Is that today the best therapeutic option for this given patient with his given prostate cancer?, and responsibility in realization: am I in the best situation to perform the optimal care. All these points are becoming prominent today because prostate cancer surgery leads to definitive side effects in patients who are not suffering from any symptoms when surgery is indicated, aiming for an hypothetical benefit in term of survival, many years down the road.

Ultimately, the responsibility of the teachers is therefore essential to highlight these questions, educate young uro-oncologists, and raise aftermath questions about surgical quality: it is with these responsibilities in mind that this chapter was written.

Beyond the technical considerations, since internships and fellowships by experienced mentors are the ultimate best way to learn surgery (in the operative room and not through medias, whatever they are) this chapter emphasizes the questions urologists should have in mind when they decide to perform a laparoscopic radical prostatectomy.

Intraoperative and Perioperative Complications

After the initial introduction of laparoscopic radical prostatectomy (LRP) [1] there was enthusiasm and hope that this technique would have a better safety profile and better functional outcomes without compromising the oncologic outcomes. Like other surgical procedures, LRP is dependent on the expertise and experience of the surgeon.

I. Sternberg, M.D. • A. Touijer, M.D.
Department of Urology, Memorial Sloan Kettering Cancer Center, New York, NY, USA

G. Maia, M.D. • B.D. Guillonneau, M.D., Ph.D., Dr. h.c. (✉)
Department of Urology, Diaconesses-Croix St. Simon Hospital, 12 rue du Sergent Bauchat, 75010 Paris, France
e-mail: bguillonneau@hopital-dcss.org

R.V. Khanna et al. (eds.), *Surgical Techniques for Prostate Cancer*,
DOI 10.1007/978-1-4939-1616-0_5, © Springer Science+Business Media New York 2015

Table 5.1 Intraoperative and perioperative complications

	RRP	LRP	
MSKCC report for 1,176 patients between 2003 and 2005 [2]	$N=692$	$N=484$	p value
Mean operating room time (min) ($n=946$)	188 (SD 41)	199 (SD 47)	<0.0005
Mean estimated blood loss (cm³) ($n=1,070$)	1,267 (SD 660)	315 (SD 186)	<0.0005
No. transfused (%)	338 (49 %)	14 (3 %)	<0.0005
Mean length of stay (days) ($n=465$)	3.3 (SD 1.2)	2.0 (SD 1.5)	<0.0005
ER return visit	75 (11 %)	75 (15.5 %)	0.02
Reoperation	3 (0.4 %)	9 (1.9 %)	0.03
No. readmitted (%) ($n=1,162$)	8 (1.2 %)	22 (4.6 %)	0.001

While the functional outcomes have not been shown to be superior to open radical prostatectomy (ORP), LRP offers the advantages of lower intraoperative blood loss, a lower rate of perioperative transfusion, and faster convalescence.

A prospective comparison of LRP and ORP performed between 2003 and 2005 at Memorial Sloan-Kettering Cancer Center (MSKCC) [2] showed that both techniques had similar rates of neurovascular bundle (NVB) preservation (88 % bilateral preservation in LRP compared to 91 % in ORP, 6 % vs. 6 % unilateral preservation, and 5 % and 3 % of bilateral NVB resection for LRP and ORP, respectively), similar rates of positive surgical margins (11 % for both surgical techniques), and a similar median number of lymph nodes retrieved (13 and 12 for LRP and ORP, respectively). The mean operative time was longer for LRP (199 min for LRP vs. 188 min for ORP), but the estimated blood loss (EBL) was significantly lower for LRP (315 mL for LRP vs. 1267 for ORP, $p<0.0005$). The hospital stay was shorter for LRP (2.0 vs. 3.3 days), but patients after LRP had a higher rate of ER visits (15 % and 11 % for LRP and ORP, respectively), higher rate of readmission (4.6 % and 1.2 % for LRP and ORP, respectively), and a higher rate of reoperation (1.9 % and 0.4 % for LRP and ORP, respectively). At a median follow-up of 1.5 years, no difference was seen in rates of biochemical recurrence (HR 0.99 for LRP vs. ORP; 95 % CI, 0.62–1.59; $p=0.9$) (Table 5.1).

Other investigators compared ORP and LRP and have reported similar results with comparable rate of positive surgical margins, comparable rates of biochemical recurrence (BCR), lower EBL, and need for transfusion in LRP-treated patients [3–5]. In a recent review of outcomes after ORP, LRP, and robot-assisted laparoscopic prostatectomy (LARP), Coelho et al. reviewed the contemporary literature from high volume centers and found mean EBLs of 951 mL and 291.5 mL in ORP and LRP, respectively. This review also showed a lower rate of transfusion needed in LRP (20.1 % and 3.5 % for ORP and LRP, respectively) [6]. While it has been recently suggested that EBL does not affect the oncologic outcome [7], this conclusion was made after analyzing the outcome of 1,567 men who underwent ORP, and thus these results do not necessarily reflect a possible advantage of lower EBL in LRP.

While magnification, better accessibility, and the antegrade surgical approach help, the collapse of venous plexuses by the positive intra-abdominal pressure is the main contributor to the lower blood loss during LRP. A temporary increase of the pneumoperitoneum pressure to 20 mmHg during transection of the dorsal vascular complex allows for tamponade and accurate venous closure.

A retrospective review of 4,592 consecutive patients treated at MSKCC with either ORP (3,458 patients) or LRP (1,134 patients) between 1999 and 2007 found a higher overall rate of both medical and surgical postoperative complications in the LRP group (8.8 % and 14.5 % rates of medical complications in ORP and LRP, respectively, and 18.7 % and 24.5 % rates of surgical complications in ORP and LRP, respectively), but a lower rate of major surgical complications (grades III–V), most of which were bladder neck contractures [8]. The lower rate of bladder neck contractures in LRP was also shown by others, as was the need for additional surgical interventions for the correction of these contractures [9].

Oncologic Outcomes

Positive Surgical Margins

A positive surgical margin (PSM) is defined as cancer cells at the inked margin of resection. A positive surgical margin at radical prostatectomy is associated to a higher risk of recurrence and has been associated with an increased risk for both local and systemic recurrence after treatment [10–12]. The goal of any surgical technique used for treatment of cancer is complete excision with negative surgical margins, extended pelvic lymph node dissection whose role is still debated thus lowering or delaying the risk of recurrence.

The rate of positive surgical margins reported in large LRP series ranges between 11 % and 26 % [2, 8, 13–15]. The rate of PSMs varies with pathologic stage and grade and ranges from 9.1 % PSM rate in patients with low risk disease to 36.8 % in a high risk group. This is comparable to previously reported rates of PSMs of 20–27 % in ORP series [16, 17] and those reported in series comparing ORP and LRP (Table 5.2).

PSMs have been shown to be associated with a higher risk of recurrence and shorter recurrence-free survival. Busch et al. recently reported that with a median follow-up of 56 months the 10-year BCR-free survival was 59.2 % vs. 82.9 % in patients with and without PSM, respectively [18]. They also found that clinical stage T2, biopsy Gleason sum >7, and higher preoperative PSA levels were all independent predictors of PSM.

Identifying the risk factors for PSMs (Table 5.3) improves the ability to decrease the percentage of patients with PSMs, and thus improves the outcome of patients. Secin et al. analyzed the preoperative and intraoperative risk factors for PSM in 407 patients treated with LRP [19]. Some of the factors associated with PSMs are well known, such as high preoperative PSA and Gleason score of 7 or more. Also shown, as known from ORP, was that lower prostate volume is a risk factor for PSMs, and that there is a trend for more PSMs on the left side for right-sided surgeons standing to the left of the patient during surgery.

An interesting association was found between the technique of NVB dissection and rate of PSMs. Results of multivariable analysis showed that dissection in the interfascial plane was associated with a fourfold increase in risk for PSMs when compared to intrafascial plane dissection. While this may be counterintuitive, as interfascial dissection is further from the prostate, this probably reflects our inaccurate preoperative assessment of extent of disease.

Table 5.2 Surgical margin analysis

Report	Publish	Number of patients	Surgeons	RRP (%)	LRP
Lepor et al. [16]	2001	1,000	Single	19.9	
Vickers et al. [17]	2010	7,765	72 (multi-institutional)	27	
Guillonneau et al. IMM [13]	2003	1,000	3		6.9 % pT2a
					18.6 % pT2b
					30 % pT3a
					34 % pT3b
Guillonneau et al. MSKCC [28]	2008	1,564	2		13 %
Touijer et al. [2]	2008	1,430	4 (2 RRP and 2 LRP)	11	11 %
Rabbani et al. [8]	2009	4,592	–	14.6	11.3 %
Eden et al. [14]	2009	1,000	Single		13.3 %
Paul et al. [15]	2010	1,115	3		5.5 % pT2a
					10 % pT2b
					33 % pT3a
					40 % pT3b
Busch et al. [31]	2012	1,845	8		29.20 %

Table 5.3 Risk factor for PSM[a] [18–22]

Risk factor for PSM
Clinical stage >T2
Gleason >7
Preop PSA level
Lower prostate volume
Surgeon side of standing[a]
Interfascial dissection of NVB[b]
Apex dissection

[a]Left side for right-sided surgeon standing on left
[b]Fourfold increase in risk

While the significance of apical PSMs, the most common site of PSMs both in ORP and LRP, and their effect on the chance of BCR are controversial [20–22], the aim in performing a prostatectomy for prostate cancer is to avoid them. Leaving the urethra to be cut last improves the anatomical orientation of the surgeon and lowers the rate of apical PSMs.

Posterolateral PSMs hold a higher risk for BCR than apical PSMs. To lower the rate of posterolateral PSMs special attention should be paid when dissection of the NVB is conducted with intent to preserve the nerves.

Pelvic Lymph Node Dissection

The presence of lymph node metastases in prostate cancer is associated with poor outcome. The most accurate way to stage the pelvic lymph nodes is by performing a pelvic lymph node dissection (PLND) at the time of prostatectomy. This allows for better identification of patients with lymph node metastases, allows for better prognostication, and improves the decision making regarding the need for further treatment. While PLND has a prognostic importance by better staging the patients, it has also been shown to have a therapeutic effect. The extent of lymph node dissection has also been shown to be important, as the more extensive a dissection is performed the higher the chances are of finding positive lymph nodes. The lymph node count has also been shown to be an objective indicator of the quality of surgery [23].

The use of prostate-specific antigen (PSA) for screening men for prostate cancer has caused a downward stage shift with an increasing number of patients diagnosed with low risk prostate cancer during the PSA screening era [24]. This has led some surgeons to omit a pelvic lymph node dissection during radical prostatectomy in men with lower risk prostate cancer. This trend found fertile ground among minimally invasive surgeons as a way to shorten surgical time.

A comparison of ORP and LRP performed at MSKCC showed a comparable number of lymph nodes extracted (12 and 13 for ORP and LRP, respectively) [2].

Other groups have reported on different criteria for performing a PLND with varying percentage of patients receiving a PLND and different percentage of patients found to have nodal metastases. The Montsouris group selected patients with cT2b, PSA > 10, and predominant Gleason pattern 4 for PLND. Of 1,000 patients, 216 (21.6 %) underwent a PLND, using these definitions, and 6 (0.6 % of the entire cohort) were found to have nodal metastases [13]. Stolzenburg et al. reported their recent experience of endoscopic extraperitoneal radical prostatectomy in which a PLND was performed on patients with PSA >10 ng/mL and/or a Gleason sum >6. This selection resulted in 1219 PLNDs (50.8 %) with metastases detected in 75 patients (6.1 %). Recently, the Henri Mondor Hospital reported oncologic outcomes based on 1,115 extraperitoneal LRPs. Limited PLNDs were performed in 75 % of the patients (those with biopsy Gleason score >6 and/or PSA >10 ng/mL), yielding a median 3.5 nodes per side and detecting lymph node metastases in 24 patients [15].

The reverse shift of stages seen among patients treated with radical prostatectomy, as more patients with low risk prostate cancer are put on active surveillance protocols [25], supports the importance of performing an extended lymph node dissection instead of omitting it. For these reasons, the MSKCC indications and anatomical template for PLND during LRP have changed from performing no lymphadenectomy for men with low risk of nodal metastases (<2 %) and a limited lymphadenectomy for those with patients with ≥2 % risk (as determined by a nomogram),

Table 5.4 Laparoscopic pelvic lymph node dissection

Report	Number of patients	Underwent PLND	Criteria	Metastases (%)	Median lymph nodes retrieved
Guillonneau et al. IMM [13]	1,000	21.6 %(216)	PSA > 10, cT2b and G 4	0.6	–
Stolzenburg et al. [26]	2,400	50.8 % (1219)	PSA > 10 or G >6	6.1	–
Paul et al. [15]	1,115	41.6 % (464)	PSA > 10 or G >6	2.2	7
Touijer et al. [27]	971	46 % (447)	Nomogram ≥2 %	14.3	13
Guillonneau et al. MSKCC [28]	1,564	58 % (828)	Nomogram >1 %	7	12

to performing an extended PLND dissection in all patients undergoing LRP. This modification has allowed retrieval of higher median nodal counts (13 [IQR 9–18] and 9 [IQR 6–13], respectively, $p < 0.001$) and increased threefold the detection of positive lymph nodes (14.3 % and 4.5 %, respectively) [27]. We concluded that a PLND including the external iliac, obturator, and hypogastric lymph node groups yields positive nodes more frequently and retrieves a higher total nodal count than the often-performed lymph node dissection limited to the external iliac nodes [28, 29] (Table 5.4).

Biochemical Recurrence

Most available data show favorable short-term and mid-term oncologic outcomes after LRP.

In a report on 1,564 consecutive patients treated with LRP in L'Institut Mutualiste Montsouris and at MSKCC, by one of two surgeons, the actuarial probabilities of remaining free of BCR at 5 and 8 years postoperatively were found to be 78 % and 71 %, respectively. The median follow-up for patients without BCR in this study was 1.5 years. The 5-year progression-free probability for men with low, moderate, and high risk prostate cancer was 91 %, 77 %, and 53 %, respectively. The 5-year progression-free probability after LRP was 83 % among patients with pathologic organ-confined disease and negative lymph nodes and 69 % among patients with pathologic non-organ-confined disease and negative lymph nodes.

In a summary of the first 1,115 LRP cases at the Hospital Henri Mondor, Paul et al. found a 3-year and 5-year recurrence-free survival rates of 84 % and 83 %, respectively [15]. Most of the patients (60 %) in this cohort had pathologic organ-confined disease, 23 % had extracapsular extension, 10 % had seminal vesical invasion, and 7 % had pathologic T4 disease. Positive lymph nodes were found in 24 (2.2 %) of patients, and 26 % of patients had PSMs. The 5-year progression-free survival rates were 93.4 %, 70.2 %, and 42.7 % for patients with pT2, pT3, and pT4 diseases.

Hruza et al. recently reported on long-term oncologic outcomes in 500 consecutive patients treated with LRP, of which 370 had complete data and were included in the analysis. Of these, 60 % had pathologic stage T2, 21 % had stage T3a, and 19 % had stage T3b/T4. Gleason 6 or less was found in 49 % of patients, while 41 % had Gleason 7, and 10 % had a Gleason sum of 8 or more. With a median follow-up of 105 months, the 10-year BCR-free survival rate was reported to be 70.6 %. When stratified according to pathologic stage, patients with pT2 had a 10-year BCF-free survival rate of 82.3 % while patients with pT3a and pT3b/pT4 diseases had a 10-year BCR-free survival rate of 54.1 % and 52.8 %, respectively [30].

Busch et al. also reported on long-term oncologic outcomes of 1,845 evaluable patients treated with LRP. With a median follow-up of 56 months, a 10-year overall survival rate of 92.5 % and a 10-year BCR-free rate of 75.6 % were found. This cohort included 50 % of patients with low risk disease, 39 % with intermediate risk, and

Table 5.5 Biochemical recurrence

Report	Number of patients	Progression-free stratified risk			Global BCR-free (%)	Time after surgery (years)
Guillonneau et al. [28]	1,564	Low	91 %		78	5
		Int.	77 %			
		High	53 %			
Paul et al. [15]	1,115	pT2	93.4 %		83	5
		pT3	70.2 %			
		pT4	42.7 %			
Hruza et al. [30]	370	pT2	82.3 %		70.6	10
		pT3	54.1 %			
		pT4	52.8 %			
Busch et al. [31]	1,845	Low	1.00	HR	75.6	10
		Int.	2.03			
		High	3.81			

11 % with high risk disease according to D'Amico's risk groups [31] (Table 5.5).

Functional Outcomes

In addition to cancer control, patients with prostate cancer are concerned about functional outcomes after treatment. The main concerns are regarding continence and erectile function and their impact on quality of life, acknowledging that infertility is constant and that sperm banking should be offered to all patients prior to any surgery.

Continence

Urinary incontinence is a bothersome problem after prostatectomy. It has many implications, both social and personal, and is a major contributor to lower quality of life after surgery. Several preoperative measures have been identified to predict postoperative continence, including age, prostate volume, urethral length, BMI, and comorbidities. A previous transurethral resection of the prostate (TURP) has also been implicated as a risk factor for post-prostatectomy incontinence (Table 5.6).

While it is hard to summarize the continence rates after LRP because of different continence definitions used in the different reports and the reporting of continence at different time points

Table 5.6 Incontinence risk factors

Incontinence risk factors
Age
Prostate volume
Urethral length
BMI
Comorbidities
TURP

after LRP (Table 5.1), overall the continence rates after LRP are good and comparable to previously reported continence rate after ORP.

Ploussard et al. looked at continence rates in 911 patients treated with LRP, who prospectively completed self-administered questionnaires, using a strict definition of no urine leak or pad use. They found that 94.4 % and 97.4 % were continent 1 and 2 years after surgery, respectively, using these strict definitions [32].

Busch el al. reported on a 74.9 % rate of continence after LRP in a cohort of 1,845 patients with a median follow-up of 56 months. They used a definition of the need for 0–1 pads per day [31].

Eden et al. reviewed their first 1,000 cases of LRP for cT1-3 prostate cancer and found that while only 10 % of patients were continent at the time of catheter removal after surgery, the pad-free rate increased to 94.9 % at a median follow-up of 27.7 months [14] (Table 5.7).

The effect of a previous TURP on continence after LRP has recently been evaluated by several

Table 5.7 Continence rates after laparoscopic radical prostatectomy

Report	Number of patients	Definition of continence	Time after surgery	Rate of continence (%)
Ploussard et al. [32]	911	No pads	12 months	94.40
			24 months	97.40
Busch et al. [31]	1,845	0–1 pads/24 h	Median f/u 56 months	74.90
Eden et al. [14]	1,000	No pads	Catheter removal	10
			Median f/u 27.7 months	94.90
Galli et al. [50]	150	"Completely continent"	Catheter removal	44.30
			12 months	91.70
Guillonneau et al. [51]	255	ICS questionnaire	12 months	82.30
Goeman et al. [52]	550	"No pads and no leakage"	1 month	38
			12 months	82.90
			24 months	90.90

groups [33, 34]. Teber et al. reported on 55 patients treated with LRP for prostate cancer found on TURP and compared them to a matched cohort of 55 patients treated by LRP for prostate cancer detected by transrectal ultrasound-guided prostate biopsies. The continence rate at 3 months after surgery was significantly lower in the first group (49.1 % vs. 61.8 %, $p = 0.01$). However the continence rates at 12 and 24 months were not statistically different. At 24 months after surgery continence rates of 92.8 % and 94.5 % were seen in patients after TURP and those not after TURP, respectively. This comparison also found a similar rate of anastomotic strictures in these groups (3.6 % and 1.8 %, respectively, $p = 0.9$). Menard et al. also found a similar rate of continence 24 months after surgery (86.9 % and 95.8 % in patients with and without previous TURP, respectively). This report found a statistically significant higher rate of anastomotic strictures in patients treated with LRP after TURP (6.5 % and 1.2 %, respectively, $p = 0.02$).

Technical Points to Improve Continence

Transection of the dorsal vascular complex without prior ligation, using the tamponade effect of the pneumoperitoneum, allows for a more accurate transection following the contour of the anterior aspect of the prostate. After transection is completed, and clear margins are assured, the pneumoperitoneum can be lowered to the usual pressure and each vein can be sutured separately. Using this technique allows for diminished disruption of the anterior sphincter complex, the width of the complex is left unchanged and relationship to the urethra is maintained. Because of the division of the puboprostatic ligaments close to the prostate and preservation of the apical aspects of the endopelvic fascia, the anterior aspect of the anastomosis is left suspended by these ligaments, the anatomical position of the vesicourethral anastomosis remains identical as for normal female anatomy.

Erectile Function

The preservation of erectile function is often a concern among patients diagnosed with localized prostate cancer considering the different treatment options. Since the introduction of nerve-sparing prostatectomy, its efficacy has been acknowledged for potency recovery and its positive role in continence has also been established. Therefore, nerve-sparing surgery has become the standard approach in all patients when oncologically possible, without compromising the oncologic outcome [35, 36] when correctly performed.

LRP was introduced with an aim to improve functional outcomes, while maintaining adequate oncologic control. The understanding of the different fascial planes of NVB dissection helped perform different degrees of nerve-sparing surgery. Adjusting the plane of dissection to the extent of disease minimizes the risk of PSMs and maximizes the potential for cavernous nerves preservation. Additionally, a high rate of accessory pudendal arteries has been identified [37]. The preservation of the majority of these accessory arteries can be accomplished without compromising the oncologic outcome [38].

Salomon et al. reported on 235 consecutive men treated with LRP for localized prostate cancer. Urinary continence and erectile function were assessed in all patients using a questionnaire derived from the ICS-male questionnaire. The questionnaire was administered preoperatively and 1, 3, 6, and 12 months postoperatively. At the time of their report, 100 consecutive men completed all questionnaires. Among patients with good preoperative erectile function who had bilateral preservation of the NVB the potency rate at 12 months was 58.8 %. Patients with unilateral NVB preservation or bilateral NVB excision had potency rates of 53.8 % and 38.4 % at 1 year, respectively [39].

Su et al. described a combined retrograde and antegrade laparoscopic approach to NVB dissection during LRP and reported their experience with 177 men treated with this technique [40]. On the basis of their experience 76 % of men sexually active and treated with this technique were reported the ability to engage in sexual intercourse 12 months after surgery. Potency was defined as the ability to achieve an erection sufficient for penetration and intercourse with or without sildenafil citrate.

A recent report by Taniguchi et al. evaluated the erectile function outcome of 27 Japanese men treated with LRP [41]. The evaluation of the erectile function included a subjective assessment by administering two questionnaires (International Index of Erection Function and Erection Hardness Score questionnaires) and an objective assessment of the rigidity and tumescence with a RigiScan in response to audiovisual stimulation. The assessment was done before surgery and at 3, 6, and 12 months after surgery. At 12 months after surgery the subjective erectile function was almost half that of the preoperative one, while the objective assessment showed rigidity of 92.6 %

and 96.3 % at the tip and base of the penis, respectively, 1 year after surgery compared to baseline preoperative rigidity. Recovery rates of penile tumescence from baseline at 1 year were 87 % at tip and 76 % at base. The discrepancy between the objective outcomes and the subjective perception of patients could be explained by the low percentage of patients in this study who had sexual intercourse during the 12 months after surgery (33 %). An additional explanation offered by the authors is a cultural feature of Japanese men who underestimate self-potency. In either case, this study shows the difficulty of assessing potency after surgery even when validated questionnaires are used.

In a prospective comprehensive comparative analysis of LRP and ORP performed by experienced surgeons at MSKCC from 2003 to 2005, Touijer et al. reported a comparable extent of NVB preservation between surgery groups: 88 % and 91 % for bilateral preservation, 6 % and 6 % for the unilateral preservation, and 5 % and 3 % for the bilateral NVB resection rate ($p = 0.2$) for the LRP and ORP groups, respectively. At 12 months postoperatively, the recovery of sexual function was also comparable between LRP and ORP during the study period. With adjustment for age and nerve-sparing status, there was no significant difference in the recovery of postoperative potency by technique (HR 1.04 for LRP vs. ORP [95 % CI, 0.74–1.46; $p = 0.8$]) [2].

Roumeguere et al. compared the erectile function outcome of patients treated with either ORP or LRP using questions 3 ("How often were you able to obtain an erection to be able to penetrate your partner?") and 4 ("How often were you able to maintain your erection after you had penetrated your partner?") of the International Index of Erectile Function questionnaire and found similar rates of postoperative potency at 1 year (54.5 % and 65.3 % for ORP and LRP, respectively) [42] (Table 5.8).

The introduction of the laparoscopic approach to radical prostatectomy was accompanied by hope that the magnification, better anatomical visualization, and lower blood loss would translate into better preservation of the NVB and better erectile function outcomes. To date, the

Table 5.8 Erection function rates 12 months after laparoscopic radical prostatectomy

Report	No. patients	Bilateral NVB (%)	Unilateral NVB	No preservation (%)
Salomon et al. [39]	100	58.8	53.8 %	38.4
Su et al. [40]	177	76	–	–
Taniguchi et al. [41][a]	27	87–76	Similar to bil.	–
Goeman et al. [52]	550	64	20.7 %	–
Guillonneau et al. [2]	81	78	–	–
Roumeguere et al. [42]	26	65.3	–	–

[a]Tumescence RigiScan

superiority of LRP in preservation of erectile function has not been proven, but has been shown to be similar to that of ORP.

Trifecta

The combination of oncologic control and a favorable functional outcome is the aim of surgery for prostate cancer. The combination of complete excision of the prostate without BCR and a good functional outcome (potency and continence) has been coined together and termed "trifecta." Trifecta has been used to assess the optimal outcome of patients treated for clinically localized prostate cancer.

Ploussard et al. assessed the oncologic and functional outcomes in 911 consecutive patients treated with LRP and who were continent and potent before surgery [32]. Urinary continence was defined as no use of pads. Potency was defined as the ability to achieve an erection sufficient for penetration with or without the use of PDE5 inhibitors. Two years after surgery 13.3 % of patients had experienced BCR, 97.4 % of patients were continent, and 64.6 % of patients were potent. At 2 years trifecta outcome was achieved 54.4 % of patients.

Although comparison of these two reports cannot be done due to possible difference in case mix, Bianco et al. reported a trifecta rate of 60 % 2 years after ORP [43]. With a median follow-up time of 6 years, 83 % of patients were free of BCR in this report, the actuarial continence recovery probability at 24 months was 95 % and the estimated recovery of potency was 70 % at 24 months in this cohort.

Salvage Laparoscopic RP

BCR after radiotherapy for prostate cancer can be secondary to local recurrent or persistent disease or metastatic disease. A select group of patient with local disease, proven by a prostate biopsy, will benefit from a salvage prostatectomy.

The BCR-free probability 5 years after a salvage prostatectomy was recently reported to be 48 % in a multi-institutional collaborative report of salvage radical prostatectomies for radiation-recurrent prostate cancer [44]. Of 404 patients included in this report 25 % had PSM, 30 % had seminal vesical invasion, and 16 % had lymph node metastases. At a median follow-up of 4.4 years, 195 experienced BCR, 64 developed metastases, and 40 patients died of prostate cancer.

Vallancien et al. were the first to report their experience with laparoscopic salvage prostatectomy [45]. The mean operative time report was 190 min, the EBL was 50–1,100 mL, and no patient was transfused. There were no conversions to open surgery and the average postoperative hospital stay was 6.4 days. At a mean follow-up of 11.2 months five of seven patients were free of BCR, five patients were continent, and all patients were impotent.

Table 5.9 BCR-free after salvage prostatectomy

Report	No. patients	Time	PSM (%)	BCR-free (%)	Continence (%)	Potency (%)
Chad et al. [44]	404	5 years	25	48	–	–
Vallencien et al. [45]	7	11.2 months	28.5	71	100	0
Liatsikos [46]	12	20 months	50	92	83	0
Ahallal et al. [47]	15	12 months	13	73	46	6.70

Since this first report a few additional small series were published. Liatsikos et al. reported on 12 patients treated with salvage LRP after failure of high intensity focused ultrasound (HIFU) or radiotherapy [46]. A mean operative time of 153 min, average EBL of 238 mL, and no need for transfusions were reported. PSM were found in 50 % of patients with a pathologic stage T3 and 12.5 % of those with a pathologic stage T2 (Table 5.9). At a mean follow-up time of 20 months one patient experienced BCR 12 months after surgery. Ten of 12 patients were continent after surgery, while 2 patients needed 1–2 pads per day. All patients were impotent after surgery (three reported on good erectile function before salvage LRP).

The MIS urology group at MSKCC reported their experience on 25 patients on 15 patients treated with salvage LRP after failure of external beam radiation (8 patients), brachytherapy (6 patients) or cryotherapy (1 patient) [47]. There were no perioperative mortalities, no conversions to open surgery, and the mean operative time was 235 min. The median EBL was 200 mL and none of the patients received transfusion. One patient had an intraoperative rectal injury that was primarily repaired and protected with a diverting colostomy, hospital stay was 2–8 days and the average length of urethral catheter was 15 days. The median number of lymph nodes removed at surgery was 16, and 2 of 15 patients had lymph node metastases. Eleven of 13 patients without lymph node metastases were free of BCR at a median follow-up of 8 months. Three patients had persistent PSA after surgery and a fourth patient experienced BCR 21 months after surgery. Seven patients achieved continence at a median time of 8.4 months after surgery and one patient had severe stress incontinence and underwent a successful implantation of an artificial urethral sphincter. The remaining seven patients continued to need 1–2 pads per day at a median follow-up time of 12.6 months after surgery. Erectile dysfunction was present in five patients preoperatively and only one patient could achieve erections after surgery.

Learning Curve

As with any surgical procedure surgeons with more LRP experience have better outcomes. Assessing the learning curve of a surgical procedure necessitates defining an end point by which the improvement will be judged. Most reports on the learning curve of LRP utilized the operative time, EBL, and functional outcomes to assess the improvement in surgical technique with growing numbers of patients treated, while others used the oncologic outcome as the end point used to assess improvement. The use of oncologic outcomes as the end point is compromised by the change in patient characteristics, as an experienced surgeon is more likely to treat patients with higher risk cancer than less experienced surgeons.

Eden et al. reported on their first 1,000 LRP cases. The learning curve was assessed using the operative time, EBL, complication rate, and functional outcome [14]. They found that while the learning curve for operative time and EBL was overcome after 100–150 cases, the learning curve for complication rate and continence took 150–200 cases and the learning curve for erectile function preservation stabilized only after 700 cases. The authors noted that there are different learning curves for LRP which are dependent on the volume of surgical procedures in the department where the procedure is taught. They recommended that LRP not be self taught and that a large surgical volume is probably needed for teaching LRP.

Table 5.10 Learning curve

Report	No. patients	PSM	BCR-free	Continence	Potency	Operative time	EBL
Eden et al. [14]	1,000	–	–	150–200	700	100–150	100–150
Secin et al. [48]	9,336	200–250	–	–	–	–	–
Vickers et al. [49]	4,702	–	750	–	–	–	–

In an international multicenter study assessing the learning curve of LRP Secin et al. used the rate of PSM as the end point for calculating the learning curve [48]. The study cohort included 9,336 patients with clinically localized prostate cancer treated with LRP by 1 of 51 surgeons in 1 of 14 institutes in North America and Europe. Forty-three percent of surgeons included performed less than 50 previous LRPs while 49 % performed at least 100 procedures. Fifty-six percent of patients included were treated by a surgeon who had performed less than 250 previous LRPs while 44 % of patients were treated by a surgeon who had performed 250 or more prior LRPs. Overall, PSMs were reported in 22 % of patients (14 % in patients with organ-confined disease and 42 % in patients with non-organ-confined disease). After controlling for case mix, they found that the rate of PSMs plateaued after 200–250 cases.

Vickers et al. assessed the learning curve for LRP, using BCR as an end point, among 29 surgeons in 7 institutes in North America and Europe [49]. Forty-one percent of surgeons included in this report had a lifetime experience of less than 50 LRP procedures, 7 % had a lifetime experience of 50–99 procedures, 34 % had a lifetime experience of 100–250 procedures, and 17 % of surgeons had a lifetime experience of more than 250 LRP procedures. Thirteen of 29 (45 %) surgeons had no previous experience with ORP while 10 % performed more than 250 ORP procedures before their first laparoscopic procedure. The 5-year BCR-free probability in this cohort was 82 %. In a model adjusted for case mix, greater surgeon experience was associated with a lower probability of recurrence ($p = 0.0053$). The risk of recurrence at 5 years decreases from 17 % for surgeons with 10 previous LRPs to 16 % among surgeons with 250 previous LRPs and to 9 % among surgeons with 750 previous LRPs (Table 5.10). In a multivariable model adjusting

for case mix they found that surgeon with previous open RP experience correlated with poorer outcome when performing LRP ($p = 0.014$).

Conclusion

Surgeons involved in prostate cancer surgery harbor a wide responsibility, not only in performing surgery without immediate complications but at first in deciding the correct indication as well. Experience in radial prostatectomy has a major impact on oncologic and functional outcomes, whatever the approach selected, retropubic, conventional laparoscopy, or with robotic assistance. It is not acceptable to focus on artificial end points, and recognizing the difficulty of such procedure is the best way to seek for improvements. Internships and fellowships are indispensable to shorten and accelerate the learning curve, in full knowledge of the risks associated with this surgery.

References

1. Guillonneau B, et al. Laparoscopic radical prostatectomy: technical and early oncological assessment of 40 operations. Eur Urol. 1999;36(1):14–20.
2. Touijer K, et al. Comprehensive prospective comparative analysis of outcomes between open and laparoscopic radical prostatectomy conducted in 2003 to 2005. J Urol. 2008;179(5):1811–7. discussion 1817.
3. Schmeller N, Keller H, Janetschek G. Head-to-head comparison of retropubic, perineal and laparoscopic radical prostatectomy. Int J Urol. 2007;14(5):402–5.
4. Rassweiler J, et al. Laparoscopic versus open radical prostatectomy: a comparative study at a single institution. J Urol. 2003;169(5):1689–93.
5. Park S, et al. Contemporary laparoscopic and open radical retropubic prostatectomy: pathologic outcomes and Kattan postoperative nomograms are equivalent. Urology. 2007;69(1):118–22.
6. Coelho RF, et al. Retropubic, laparoscopic, and robot-assisted radical prostatectomy: a critical review

of outcomes reported by high-volume centers. J Endourol. 2010;24(12):2003–15.

7. Djavan B, et al. Blood loss during radical prostatectomy: impact on clinical, oncological and functional outcomes and complication rates. BJU Int. 2012;110(1):69–75.

8. Rabbani F, et al. Comprehensive standardized report of complications of retropubic and laparoscopic radical prostatectomy. Eur Urol. 2010;57(3):371–86.

9. Wagner AA, et al. Comparison of open and laparoscopic radical prostatectomy outcomes from a surgeon's early experience. Urology. 2007;70(4):667–71.

10. Catalona WJ, Smith DS. Cancer recurrence and survival rates after anatomic radical retropubic prostatectomy for prostate cancer: intermediate-term results. J Urol. 1998;160(6 Pt 2):2428–34.

11. Kattan MW, Wheeler TM, Scardino PT. Postoperative nomogram for disease recurrence after radical prostatectomy for prostate cancer. J Clin Oncol. 1999;17(5):1499–507.

12. Stamey TA, et al. Biological determinants of cancer progression in men with prostate cancer. JAMA. 1999;281(15):1395–400.

13. Guillonneau B, et al. Laparoscopic radical prostatectomy: oncological evaluation after 1,000 cases a Montsouris Institute. J Urol. 2003;169(4):1261–6.

14. Eden CG, Neill MG, Louie-Johnsun MW. The first 1000 cases of laparoscopic radical prostatectomy in the UK: evidence of multiple 'learning curves'. BJU Int. 2009;103(9):1224–30.

15. Paul A, et al. Oncologic outcome after extraperitoneal laparoscopic radical prostatectomy: midterm follow-up of 1115 procedures. Eur Urol. 2010;57(2): 267–72.

16. Lepor H, Nieder AM, Ferrandino MN. Intraoperative and postoperative complications of radical retropubic prostatectomy in a consecutive series of 1,000 cases. J Urol. 2001;166(5):1729–33.

17. Vickers A, et al. The learning curve for surgical margins after open radical prostatectomy: implications for margin status as an oncological end point. J Urol. 2010;183(4):1360–5.

18. Busch J, et al. Impact of positive surgical margins on oncological outcome following laparoscopic radical prostatectomy (LRP): long-term results. World J Urol. 2013;31(2):395–401.

19. Secin FP, et al. Preoperative and intraoperative risk factors for side-specific positive surgical margins in laparoscopic radical prostatectomy for prostate cancer. Eur Urol. 2007;51(3):764–71.

20. Kordan Y, et al. Impact of positive apical surgical margins on likelihood of biochemical recurrence after radical prostatectomy. J Urol. 2009;182(6):2695–701.

21. Pettus JA, et al. Biochemical failure in men following radical retropubic prostatectomy: impact of surgical margin status and location. J Urol. 2004;172(1):129–32.

22. Stephenson AJ, et al. Location, extent and number of positive surgical margins do not improve accuracy of predicting prostate cancer recurrence after radical prostatectomy. J Urol. 2009;182(4):1357–63.

23. Mazzola C, et al. Nodal counts during pelvic lymph node dissection for prostate cancer: an objective indicator of quality under the influence of very subjective factors. BJU Int. 2012;109(9):1323–8.

24. Cooperberg MR, et al. Time trends in clinical risk stratification for prostate cancer: implications for outcomes (data from CaPSURE). J Urol. 2003;170 (6 Pt 2):S21–5; discussion S26-7.

25. Silberstein JL, et al. Reverse stage shift at a tertiary care center: escalating risk in men undergoing radical prostatectomy. Cancer. 2011;117(21):4855–60.

26. Stolzenburg JU, et al. Endoscopic extraperitoneal radical prostatectomy: evolution of the technique and experience with 2400 cases. J Endourol. 2009;23 (9):1467–72.

27. Touijer K, et al. Extending the indications and anatomical limits of pelvic lymph node dissection for prostate cancer: improved staging or increased morbidity? BJU Int. 2011;108(3):372–7.

28. Touijer K, et al. Oncologic outcome after laparoscopic radical prostatectomy: 10 years of experience. Eur Urol. 2009;55(5):1014–9.

29. Touijer K, et al. Standard versus limited pelvic lymph node dissection for prostate cancer in patients with a predicted probability of nodal metastasis greater than 1 %. J Urol. 2007;178(1):120–4.

30. Hruza M, et al. Long-term oncological outcomes after laparoscopic radical prostatectomy. BJU Int. 2013; 111(2):271–80.

31. Busch J, et al. Long-term oncological and continence outcomes after laparoscopic radical prostatectomy: a single-centre experience. BJU Int. 2012;110 (11 Pt C):E985–90.

32. Ploussard G, et al. Prospective evaluation of combined oncological and functional outcomes after laparoscopic radical prostatectomy: trifecta rate of achieving continence, potency and cancer control at 2 years. BJU Int. 2011;107(2):274–9.

33. Menard J, et al. Laparoscopic radical prostatectomy after transurethral resection of the prostate: surgical and functional outcomes. Urology. 2008;72(3): 593–7.

34. Teber D, et al. Laparoscopic radical prostatectomy in clinical T1a and T1b prostate cancer: oncologic and functional outcomes—a matched-pair analysis. Urology. 2009;73(3):577–81.

35. Eggleston JC, Walsh PC. Radical prostatectomy with preservation of sexual function: pathological findings in the first 100 cases. J Urol. 1985;134(6):1146–8.

36. Walsh PC, Mostwin JL. Radical prostatectomy and cystoprostatectomy with preservation of potency. Results using a new nerve-sparing technique. Br J Urol. 1984;56(6):694–7.

37. Secin FP, et al. Anatomy of accessory pudendal arteries in laparoscopic radical prostatectomy. J Urol. 2005;174(2):523–6; discussion 526.

38. Secin FP, et al. Positive surgical margins and accessory pudendal artery preservation during laparoscopic radical prostatectomy. Eur Urol. 2005;48(5):786–92; discussion 793.

39. Salomon L, et al. Urinary continence and erectile function: a prospective evaluation of functional results after radical laparoscopic prostatectomy. Eur Urol. 2002;42(4):338–43.
40. Su LM, et al. Nerve-sparing laparoscopic radical prostatectomy: replicating the open surgical technique. Urology. 2004;64(1):123–7.
41. Taniguchi H, et al. Recovery of erectile function after nerve-sparing laparoscopic radical prostatectomy in Japanese patients undergoing both subjective and objective assessments. J Sex Med. 2012;9(7):1931–6.
42. Roumeguere T, et al. Radical prostatectomy: a prospective comparison of oncological and functional results between open and laparoscopic approaches. World J Urol. 2003;20(6):360–6.
43. Bianco Jr FJ. P.T. Scardino, and J.A. Eastham, Radical prostatectomy: long-term cancer control and recovery of sexual and urinary function ("trifecta"). Urology. 2005;66(5 Suppl):83–94.
44. Chade DC, et al. Salvage radical prostatectomy for radiation-recurrent prostate cancer: a multi-institutional collaboration. Eur Urol. 2011;60(2):205–10.
45. Vallancien G, et al. Initial results of salvage laparoscopic radical prostatectomy after radiation failure. J Urol. 2003;170(5):1838–40.
46. Liatsikos E, et al. Treatment of patients after failed high intensity focused ultrasound and radiotherapy for localized prostate cancer: salvage laparoscopic extraperitoneal radical prostatectomy. J Endourol. 2008;22(10):2295–8.
47. Ahallal Y, et al. Pilot study of salvage laparoscopic prostatectomy for the treatment of recurrent prostate cancer. BJU Int. 2011;108(5):724–8.
48. Secin FP, et al. The learning curve for laparoscopic radical prostatectomy: an international multicenter study. J Urol. 2010;184(6):2291–6.
49. Vickers AJ, et al. The surgical learning curve for laparoscopic radical prostatectomy: a retrospective cohort study. Lancet Oncol. 2009;10(5):475–80.
50. Galli S, et al. Oncologic outcome and continence recovery after laparoscopic radical prostatectomy: 3 years' follow-up in a "second generation center". Eur Urol. 2006;49(5):859–65.
51. Guillonneau B, et al. Laparoscopic radical prostatectomy: assessment after 550 procedures. Crit Rev Oncol Hematol. 2002;43(2):123–33.
52. Goeman L, et al. Long-term functional and oncological results after retroperitoneal laparoscopic prostatectomy according to a prospective evaluation of 550 patients. World J Urol. 2006;24(3):281–8.

Robotic Prostatectomy

6

Rakesh V. Khanna

Introduction

Prostate cancer is the most commonly diagnosed cancer among men in the United States of America. Radical prostatectomy is the most common treatment for localized prostate cancer. The goals of radical prostatectomy are to achieve cancer control, maintain continence, and preserve potency.

Since its introduction in 1999, the da Vinci Surgical System (Intuitive Surgical, Sunnyvale, CA) has become an integral tool in urologic surgery. Robot assistance reduced many of the challenges associated with laparoscopic prostatectomy with the result that Robot-assisted radical prostatectomy was rapidly adopted for the treatment of localized prostate cancer. Currently, more than 75 % of radical prostatectomies are performed robotically.

Advantages of the robotic system include improved ergonomics, wristed instrumentation, and magnified, three-dimensional visualization facilitating suturing and dissection during minimally invasive prostatectomy.

The robotic system consists of three components: the Surgeon Console, Patient Side Cart, and Video Tower. A dedicated robotic team aids in improving surgical efficiency while an assistant skilled in minimally invasive and robotic surgery is important in achieving optimal outcomes in robotic prostatectomy.

Robotic Prostatectomy Technique

Instruments:
Curved Monopolar Scissors
Bipolar forcep
Prograsp forcep
Suction/Irrigator
Needle Driver
Small bowel grasper
Hemolock clips and applier
Optional:
Harmonic Scalpel

Patient Positioning

After induction of general anesthesia, sequential compression devices are placed on both legs. The patient is then placed in lithotomy position with the arms tucked and padded at the patient's sides. The patient is secured to the bed and the operative table is placed in extreme Trendelenberg position as a stress test to ensure that the patient has been adequately secured.

The patient is then prepped and draped in a sterile fashion. A urethral catheter is placed and

R.V. Khanna, M.D. (✉)
Department of Urology, SUNY Upstate
Medical University, 750 East Adams Street,
Syracuse, NY 13210, USA
e-mail: khannara@upstate.edu

positioned for easy access by the assistant. A nasogastric tube is placed to decompress the stomach.

Port Placement

A 5-6-port technique is employed. The initial 12 mm trocar is placed at or just superior to the umbilicus. This will serve as the robotic camera port and as the specimen extraction site. Pneumoperitoneum is obtained using a veress needle or an open technique. Insufflation is set to 20 mmHg for port placement and then decreased to 15 mmHg for the remainder of the case. After insertion of the initial 12 mm trocar, a diagnostic laparoscopy is performed to ensure that no vascular or bowel injury has occurred. The remaining ports are then positioned under direct vision. The following 8 mm ports are positioned along a line 2 fingerbreaths below the umbilicus: the port for the right robotic arm is placed just lateral to the right rectus muscle, the port for the left robotic arm just lateral to the left rectus muscle, and the port for the third robotic arm above the left anterior superior iliac spine. Ideally the robotic ports should be separated by 8–9 cm to minimize clashing of the robotic arms. A 12-mm assistant

port is placed 2 fingerbreaths above the right anterior iliac spine and if desired another 5 mm port can be placed between the camera port and right robotic arm but 5 cm cranially. In obese patients consideration should be given to using longer ports, whereas in very tall patients port position should be displaced inferiorly (Fig. 6.1).

The patient is then placed in extreme trendelenburg position. The robot is brought in and docked between the patient's legs (Fig. 6.2). The assistant works from the patient's right side.

Developing Space of Retzius

Visualization is initially performed with a 0° endoscope. Dissection is performed with curved monopolar scissors in the right robotic arm and bipolar forcep in the left robotic arm. The fourth robotic arm controls a grasper, such as a Prograsp forcep, and is used for grasping and retracting tissues.

To retract bowel from the surgical field and to help expose the lymph node packets, adhesions between the bowel and peritoneum are released. This most commonly is required on the left side where the sigmoid colon is released from the lateral peritoneum.

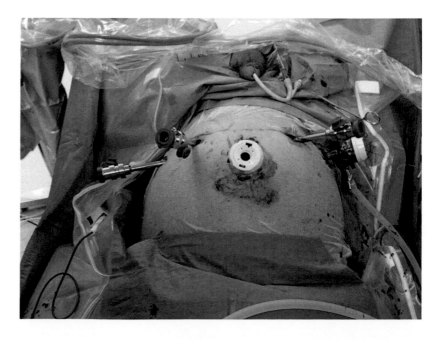

Fig. 6.1 Port position

Fig. 6.2 Docking of robot

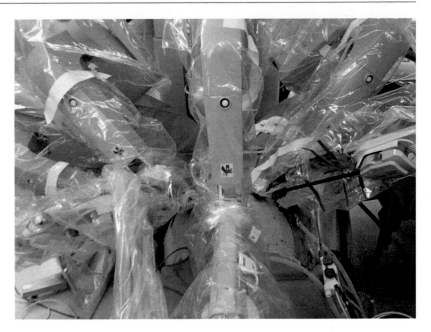

After transperitoneal access, the space of Retzius is developed and the dissection performed by an anterior technique. The bladder is dissected from the anterior abdominal wall by incising the peritoneum lateral to the medial umbilical ligaments. This incision is carried superiorly to the level of the umbilicus and inferolaterally to the level of the Vas Deferens. Care should be taken to avoid injury to the inferior epigastric vessels, which can cause troublesome bleeding or to carrying the dissection too far laterally in which case inadvertent entry into the iliac vessels may occur. The urachus is divided high above the bladder thus avoiding the presence of unnecessary tissue obstructing the field of view.

The plane between the bladder and anterior abdominal wall is then developed using a combination of blunt and sharp dissection. The correct plane is composed of fibrofatty tissue and is relatively avascular. Posterior traction on the bladder with the fourth robotic arm helps to correctly identify this tissue plane. If one is in the correct plane, one should see the pubic bone anteriorly. This dissection is continued inferiorly until the Endopelvic fascia is identified. Mobilization of the bladder is a key step in prostatectomy as it allows for a tension-free urethrovesical anastomosis to be performed.

The preceding technique, the Anterior Transperitoneal, is the most common approach to robotic prostatectomy. Another approach is the Transperitoneal Retrovesical approach in which the seminal vesicles and vas deferens are dissected first followed by bladder mobilization. Alternatively, an Extraperitoneal approach is also described but tends to be less commonly performed due to the smaller working space.

Opening Endopelvic Fascia

After release and mobilization of the bladder, the fat overlying the prostate is removed. Within this tissue lies the Superficial Dorsal Vein. It will usually lie in the midline and can lead to significant bleeding if not adequately coagulated.

At this point the endopelvic fascia and puboprostatic ligaments should be visible. Starting on the right side, the prostate is retracted medially. Opening of the endopelvic fascia is performed athermally using scissors towards the base of the prostate where the prostate is more mobile. This incision is then carried towards the apex of the prostate. The levator fibers are gently pushed away from the lateral and apical portions of the prostate (Fig. 6.3). The correct plane is avascular.

Fig. 6.3 Opening of endopelvic fascia

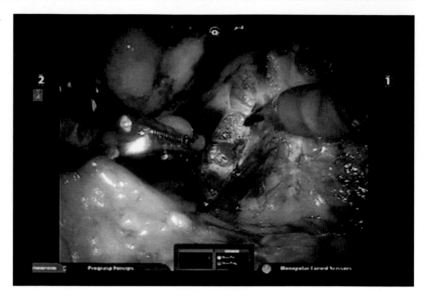

If bleeding is encountered this raises the possibility that one is dissecting through the levator
fibers.

Towards the apex of the prostate, the puboprostatic ligaments are divided. In this area, the
levator fibers may coalesce into a band of tissue
requiring sharp dissection to free up the apical
prostate.

The apical dissection proceeds until one iden-
tifies a notch between the dorsal venous complex
anteriorly and the urethra posteriorly. A similar
procedure is then repeated on the left side.

When excising the periprostatic fat or opening
the endopelvic fascia, an Accessory Pudendal
Artery may be encountered. When possible these
arteries should be preserved. These may arise laterally coursing along the prostate, coursing above
or below the endopelvic fascia or from an apical
location. While these appear to be entering the
prostate, they can often be dissected off the prostate using sharp dissection and bipolar cautery.
Towards the apex they are in close association
with the dorsal venous complex and prone to lead
to venous oozing. Therefore, before performing
this distal dissection, it may be wise to open the
contralateral endopelvic fascia such that in case
bleeding is encountered, one is prepared to suture
ligate the complex. Apical dissection of
Accessory Pudendal arteries proceeds until prox-

imal suture ligation of the dorsal venous complex
can be performed.

Ligation of Dorsal Venous Complex/ Anterior Urethra Suspension

Various techniques have been described to control the dorsal venous complex. The complex can
be suture-ligated with a 0-PDS suture on a CT-1
needle. The bladder is grasped with the fourth
robotic arm and placed on cephalad traction. The
notch between the dorsal venous complex and
urethra is identified. The suture is passed anterior
to the urethra (Fig. 6.4). After passage of the
suture, both ends are grasped. The assistant then
pushes the urethral catheter in/out to ensure that
the suture has not caught the catheter. A second
throw of the suture can then be performed and the
complex secured with a square knot. Alternatively,
after a single throw, a slipknot can be laid down
to control the complex.

Another technique to control the dorsal vein
involves the use of a laparoscopic stapling device.
Conversely, while some techniques advise dividing
the dorsal vein and suturing/stapling only if necessary, care should be taken in using this approach as
bleeding can obscure visualization and increase the
chance of a positive apical margin.

Fig. 6.4 Ligation of the dorsal venous complex

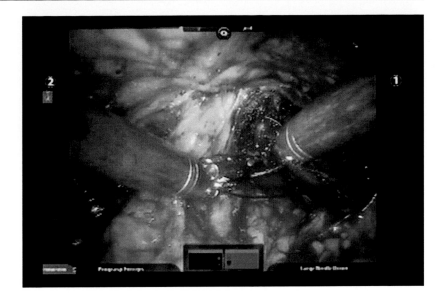

Anterior Bladder Neck

At this point it is helpful to switch to a 30° downward looking lens. While not necessary, this does help with visualization of the posterior bladder neck and during seminal vesicle dissection.

To delineate the correct plane and avoid entry into the prostate, the plane between the prostate and bladder is identified by advancing the urethral catheter in/out and applying gentle inward compression. Otherwise, the fourth arm can be used to tent the bladder anterocranially. Dissection is then initiated where the bladder tenting stops.

A horizontal incision is made in the bladder using monopolar cautery until the urethral catheter is visualized. The incision should not be made too laterally because bleeding from branches of the bladder pedicle can be encountered. The catheter balloon is then deflated and grasped by the fourth robotic arm. Simultaneously, the assistant clamps the catheter over a gauze just distal to the urethral meatus. The catheter is brought through the bladder incision and placed on cephalad retraction to elevate the prostate. Retraction can also be achieved by passing a holding suture through and through the abdominal wall, incorporating the eye of the catheter, and securing it to the outside.

Posterior Bladder Neck/Seminal Vesicle Dissection

Once the bladder is entered, the ureteral orifices are identified. In addition the presence of a median lobe should be ascertained (Fig. 6.5).

A horizontal incision is made in the posterior bladder neck using monopolar cautery. Dissection is carried at a 45° angle to avoid entry into the bladder or prostate. To avoid creation of an inadvertent cystotomy, frequent inspection of the bladder is performed.

Continuing along a 45° angle of dissection, one should identify the vasa deferentia in the midline. The depth of dissection can be estimated by considering that the thickness of the posterior bladder neck should approximate that of the anterior bladder neck. If it does not, or if the vasa deferentia are not encountered, this indicates that the plane of dissection is too superficial and may result in violation of the prostate. Furthermore, significant bleeding encountered in the midline or visualization of prostatic secretions is indicative of entry into the prostate. In each of the above cases, if one suspects entry into the prostate, one returns more cephalad and adjusts the angle of dissection more posteriorly.

If a prostate median lobe is present, division of the lateral bladder neck may be required to

Fig. 6.5 Median lobe of
the prostate. Prior to
incising the mucosa below
the median lobe, both
ureteral orifices are
identified

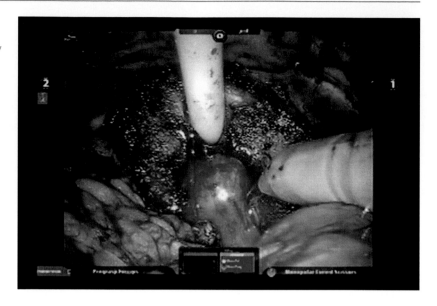

Fig. 6.5 Median lobe of the prostate. Prior to incising the mucosa below the median lobe, both ureteral orifices are identified

visualize beneath the median lobe and the posterior bladder neck. Again in the presence of a median lobe, identification of the ureteral orifices is critical. If required intravenous furosemide and indigo carmine can be administered. To aid with visualization, the median lobe is grasped with the fourth robotic arm and lifted anteriorly. Alternatively a 0 vicryl suture can be placed through the median lobe and lifted anteriorly by the assistant. Dissection must be below the median lobe as dissecting along its contour will result in incomplete resection and the vas and seminal vesicles will not be encountered.

Once the vas are identified, the fourth robotic arm releases traction on the urethral catheter and instead is used to grasp and retract the vas deferens anteriorly. Using blunt dissection the overlying tissue is released further mobilizing the vas. As the vas is lifted, this will bring up the corresponding seminal vesicle.

The arterial supply to the vas deferens typically runs between the vas and medial seminal vesicle. The vas is clipped and divided. The fourth robotic arm is repositioned to hold the proximal end and lifts anteriorly. When holding the vas, the wristed joint of the robotic instrument should be angled inferolaterally to maximize working space. Simultaneously, the assistant grasps the distal end and pulls laterally in the direction of the assistant port. This maneuver

aids in visualization and exposure of the seminal vesicles. With the seminal vesicles exposed, the vas is released. The seminal vesicle is now held and lifted anteriorly with the robotic arm angled as described previously. With the seminal vesicle on traction, blunt dissection is used to free the gland proceeding from a medial to lateral direction. The blood supply originates inferolaterally and is controlled with clips. Electrocautery should be avoided as they may result in injury to the neurovascular bundle. After one side has completed, the same procedure is performed on the remaining vas deferens and seminal vesicle.

After both seminal vesicles and vas deferens have been dissected free, they are grasped with the fourth robotic arm and lifted anteriorly to provide exposure for the posterior dissection. Alternatively, they can be grasped on one side with the fourth robotic arm and on the other side by the assistant to provide anterior traction.

An incision is then made in the midline of Denonvilliers fascia and the posterior prostatic contour is defined. A plane is created using blunt and sharp dissection between the prostate and rectum. The correct plane is identified by the visualization of perirectal fat. Dissection is continued towards the apex of the prostate and laterally to thin out the prostate pedicles. Dissection to the apex decreases the chance of rectal injury that may occur with the subsequent apical dissection.

Ligation of Vascular Pedicles

If a nerve sparing procedure is to be performed, thermal energy should be avoided due to propagation to cavernosal nerves.

It is generally easier to start with ligation of the right vascular pedicle because of the better working angles.

Different techniques exist to control the vascular pedicle. These include suture ligation, Bulldog clamps, clips, or coagulation (non-nerve sparing).

The pedicles should be adequately thinned to allow clip application. To aid with clip application, for the right prostatic pedicle the fourth robotic arm grabs the prostate and pulls it to the contralateral side while the assistant provides cephalad traction on the perivesical tissue. This puts the pedicle on stretch rendering it easier to place clips. For the left pedicle the maneuver is reversed with the assistant grabbing the prostate and the fourth robotic arm grabbing the perivesical tissue.

Alternatively, Beck described a technique of tension adjustable ligation of the vascular pedicle using a 6 cm 3-0 poliglecaprone suture on an SII needle. A figure of eight suture is placed 5–8 mm from the base of the prostate and 5–7 mm above the perirectal fat. The needle is then threaded through a preformed loop at the end of the suture. Placing a clip and cinching down on the suture ligature can then apply increasing tension on the suture.

Nerve Sparing

Nerve sparing is performed using a traction-free, athermal technique. The aggressiveness of nerve sparing should take into account a risk-stratified approach. Given that the neurovascular packets are located outside the prostatic capsule, for localized disease nerve sparing should not affect margin status provided that the capsule is not violated. In this respect, identification of patients at high risk for extracapsular extension is essential, as it would allow for the selection of patients in whom a non-nerve sparing versus a unilateral or bilateral nerve sparing procedure should be performed.

Nerve sparing is performed via an interfascial dissection. This is performed between the prostatic fascia and levator fascia laterally and Denonvilliers fascia and prostate posteriorly.

Originally considered two bundles of tissue travelling along the posterolateral surface of the prostate, the course of the neurovascular bundles has been shown to be more diffuse. The prostatic fascia is incised anterolaterally and nerve sparing proceeds towards the apex using an athermal technique (Fig. 6.6). Different terms have been used to describe this technique including the "Veil of Aphrodite" and "high anterior release."

For right-sided nerve sparing, the fourth arm is used to gently rotate the prostate medially. The prostatic fascia is incised over the anterolateral

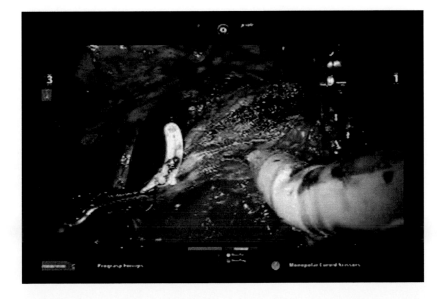

Fig. 6.6 Nerve sparing

surface. The incision is carried towards the apex in an antegrade fashion. The tissue is then released away from the prostate using sharp and blunt dissection.

Venous components are commonly the most medial component of the neurovascular bundle. This may be used as an anatomical landmark. They can be intentionally cut leaving the medial wall of the vein and the underlying inner prostatic fascia with the prostate.

To optimize potency outcomes, traction on the neurovascular bundles should be avoided. Care should also be taken to avoid incorporation of the neurovascular bundle in a suture or clip.

Compared to an Interfascial dissection, an Intrafascial dissection involves dissecting one layer closer between the prostatic fascia and capsule. This is best suited to those with low volume, low grade cancers where positive surgical margins are less likely to occur.

Apical Dissection/Transection of Urethra

At this stage of the procedure, the prostate should be free at the base, posteriorly and laterally. The only remaining attachments are the dorsal venous complex, urethra, and rectourethralis fibers.

The prostatic apex is the most common site of positive margins with radical prostatectomy.

Anatomy in this area can be highly variable and care should be taken to ensure that no lip of prostate tissue is left behind.

In this regard, optimal visualization is crucial. It is important that bleeding from the dorsal venous complex be minimal. Increasing pneumoperitoneum to 20 mmHg prior to transection of the dorsal venous complex and judicious use of suction by the assistant can help to minimize bleeding.

The base of the prostate is grasped with the third robotic arm and pulled in a cephalad direction. The dorsal venous complex is then transected using scissors (Fig. 6.7). To avoid entry into the prostate, the angle of incision should be horizontal.

After division of the complex, the urethra is visualized. It is transected a few millimeters distal to the prostatic notch (Fig. 6.8). The urethral catheter is visualized and retracted and the remaining urethra divided. The final remaining apical attachments are transected, with care taken to avoid transection of the neurovascular complex that lie in close proximity.

Traction on the prostate, directed alternatively to the patient's right and left sides, assists in delineation of the apex (Fig. 6.9).

After division of the urethra, the remaining rectourethralis fibers are divided. It is at this step that the rectum is most at risk of injury. As stated previously maximal posterior dissection to the apex

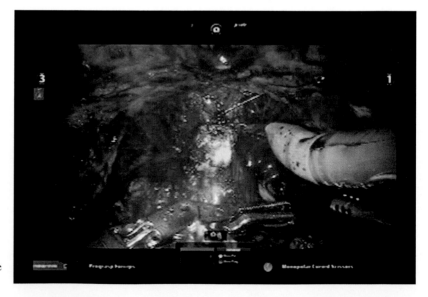

Fig. 6.7 Transection of the dorsal venous complex

Fig. 6.8 Transection of urethra. The urethra is transected a few millimeters distal to the prostatic notch. Preservation of urethral length facilitates the vesicourethral anastomosis and improves postoperative continence

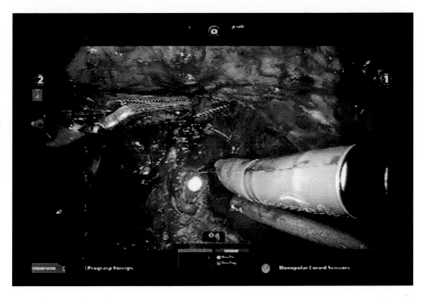

Fig. 6.9 Apical dissection. The prostate is rotated to visualize the remaining apical attachments

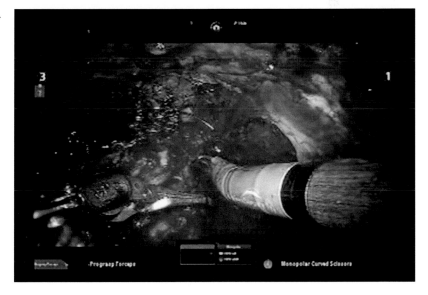

helps to decrease the chance of rectal injury. After transection of the rectourethralis fibers, the specimen is now completely free. It is inspected and if any area of concern is identified, additional sections can be sent off for frozen section analysis. The prostate is then placed in an extraction bag and stored in the abdomen for later extraction.

The neurovascular bundles appear as two tracts of tissue coursing along either side of the rectum towards the urethral stump (Fig. 6.10). The surgical site is copiously irrigated. Hemostasis is verified. Any areas of bleeding that are identified can be suture-ligated or clipped. However, care should be taken to avoid incorporating the neurovascular bundles.

Any free clips in the surgical site are removed, as they can migrate into the bladder and result in bladder calculi.

Fig. 6.10 Neurovascular bundles

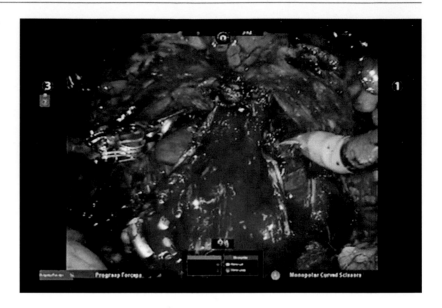

Lymph Node Dissection

If required a lymph node dissection is now performed. The extent of lymph node dissection following prostatectomy has yet to be standardized.

Tissue around the obturator nerve and along the pelvic sidewall is dissected to clear the obturator fossa. The boundary of dissection includes the External Iliac Vein anteriorly, the Pelvic side wall laterally, the femoral canal inferiorly, and the bifurcation of the Common Iliac artery superiorly. Tissue to the lateral aspect of the bladder is also cleared. If an extended lymph node dissection is to be performed, the dissection is continued proximally up to the bifurcation of the aorta.

Dissection of the right lymph node packet is generally easier due to the angle of the robotic arms. The fourth robotic arm is used to retract the bladder medially. The lymph node packet above the external iliac vein is grasped and bluntly dissected (Fig. 6.11). The vein is skeletonized. Care must be taken as often an obturator vein can be encountered and can cause significant bleeding if avulsed. The lymph node packet is carefully dissected off this vein. During dissection, clips are used on lymphatic channels to minimize development of postoperative lymphoceles.

Care must be taken to avoid injury to the obturator nerve. Prior to clip application the obturator nerve must be identified. The nerve will lie lateral to the obturator vessels. Once identified, the nerve is exposed by blunt dissection by sweeping the packet in a direction parallel to the nerve.

Vascular injuries are controlled by robotic suture ligation. Ureteral injury may occur at the proximal limit of the dissection. If any injury occurs, a stented, spatulated end to end anastomosis should be performed.

Bladder Neck/Posterior Urethral Reconstruction

In cases where an enlarged bladder neck opening is present, reconstruction can quickly be accomplished by placing figure of eight absorbable sutures at the 4 and 8 o'clock positions. If the ureteral orifices lie close to the bladder neck, ureteral stents can be placed to avoid ureteral entrapment.

While not necessary, we routinely perform a posterior reconstruction as we feel this maneuver facilitates a tension-free urethral anastomosis. Posterior reconstruction is performed by approximating Denonvilliers fascia and the posterior detrusor muscle to the posterior rhabdosphincter.

Fig. 6.11 Lymph node dissection: The lymph node packet has been dissected off the external iliac vein. The obturator nerve has been identified. The distal limit of the lymph node packet, the pubic bone, is clipped and divided

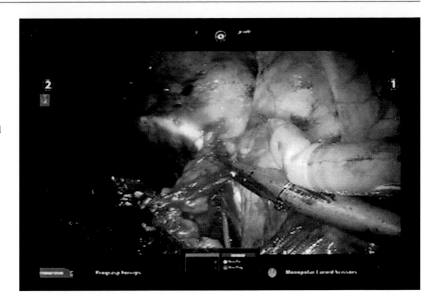

Vesico-Urethral Anastomosis

The anastomosis begins posteriorly in the midline and runs progressively anteriorly on either side. When placing sutures through the lateral portions of the urethra, care must be taken to avoid incorporation of the neurovascular bundles.

The anastomosis is performed using two eight inch 3-0 vicryl sutures that have been tied together. Alternatively, a barb suture may be used. The suture is thrown outside-in through the bladder neck and then inside-out through the urethra. After three throws have been thrown through the urethra, the surgeon pulls on the suture to cinch the bladder down to the urethra. If required, the assistant simultaneously pushes down on the bladder.

To aid with visualization of the urethral stump, switching back to a zero degree endoscope and perineal pressure applied by the assistant are effective. The assistant periodically moves the urethral catheter in/out to ensure that the urethra has not been backwalled and that the catheter itself has not been incorporated into the suture. Prior to tying down the anastomotic sutures a new 20-french urethral catheter is inserted under direct vision into the bladder.

Otherwise, a percutaneous suprapubic catheter can be placed for bladder drainage.

A watertight anastomosis is confirmed by filling the bladder with 120 cm^3 normal saline. Any areas of leakage are closed with interrupted 3-0 vicryl sutures.

A closed suction drain is placed. The robot is undocked and all ports are removed under direct vision. The specimen is extracted through the camera port.

The suction drain is removed if drainage is less than 80 cm^3/24 h or if fluid creatinine is consistent with serum levels. The catheter is left indwelling for 7–10 days. Postoperatively a cystogram in performed prior to catheter removal.

Improving Continence

Multiple technical modifications have been developed to help patients to maintain or regain continence. These modifications can generally be divided into two categories: those that limit dissection of structures supporting the urethra and posterior pelvic floor and those that reconstruct these areas after the prostate has been removed. Techniques described include bladder neck preservation, bladder neck reconstruction, preservation of urethral length, periurethral suspension, posterior reconstruction, combined anterior and posterior reconstruction, endopelvic fascia preservation, complete anterior preservation, selective suturing of the dorsal venous complex, and nerve sparing.

Preservation of natural continence mechanisms is key for patients to regain postoperative urinary control, whereas reconstructive techniques may hasten urinary recovery.

Several Described Modifications Include

Bladder Neck Preservation

The bladder neck serves as an Internal Sphincter and is composed of three distinct muscle layers including an inner longitudinal layer, a middle circular layer, and an outer longitudinal layer.

Outcomes of bladder neck preservation in open and laparoscopic series provided conflicting results with some studies showing small benefit with continence and potentially increased positive margins. However, more recent series of robotic prostatectomy have shown improved continence with no effect on positive margin rates.

Periurethral (Anterior) Suspension

After ligation of the Dorsal Venous complex, a second suture is placed through the dorsal venous complex. The suture is then passed from left to right through the pubic periosteum. The suture is then passed from right to left through the dorsal venous complex and again through the pubic periosteum and tied. This has been shown to hasten recovery of urinary incontinence at 3 months although continence at 12 months remained similar. Another advantage of this suspension is that it may decrease the chance of inadvertent transection of this suture during division of the dorsal venous complex.

Posterior Reconstruction

This reconstructs the posterior musculofascial plate. Starting on the right side, a suture is passed through the cut end of Denonvillier's fascia and posterior detrusor fibers and then through the rectourethralis fibers. This is repeated two to three times and then tied. As stated earlier, we perform this maneuver as we find it aids with a tension-free urethral anastomosis. In addition in a meta-analysis there was lower risk of postoperative urine leak. However, evidence regarding its effectiveness on urinary continence has been conflicting. Some studies have shown improvement in early return of continence with no difference in long-term continence whereas others show no benefit.

Results of studies of both combined anterior and posterior reconstruction have also been conflicting.

Selective Dorsal Venous Complex Ligation

The open venous channels are selectively ligated rather than the complex as a whole thus avoiding potential damage to surrounding levator fibers. This may lead to earlier return of continence, although long-term continence is unchanged.

Nerve Sparing

Although the rhabdosphincter receives innervation from the pudendal nerve, authors have noted an improvement in urinary continence with a nerve-sparing procedure.

Positive Margins

Most positive margins occur at the apex of the prostate. To minimize chance of apical positive margins tips include complete dissection of the fatty tissue around the puboprostatic ligaments and the dorsal venous complex, incision of the endopelvic fascia, dissection of the levator fibers from the DVC in order to increase the length of the venous plexus, and transection of the urethra 3–6 mm distal to the prostatourethral junction.

Preserving Potency

As stated earlier, the principles of nerve sparing revolve around minimal traction, athermal dissection, and dissecting within the correct tissue planes.

Nerve sparing can be performed in an antegrade fashion (base to apex) or in a retrograde fashion (apex to base).

Several techniques of nerve sparing are available including "the Veil of Aphrodite," "athermal retrograde neurovascular release," and "clipless antegrade nerve sparing."

The Veil of Aphrodite/High Anterior Release

The plane between the posterior prostatic fascia and Denonvilliers fascia is extended distally towards the apex and laterally to reveal the prostatic pedicles. The pedicles are controlled with clips. The prostatic fascia is then incised anteriorly to enter the intrafascial plane. The entire periprostatic fascia is released hanging from the pubourethral ligaments. In the Superveil modification, the dorsal venous complex and puboprostatic ligaments are also preserved.

Athermal Early Retrograde Release of the Neurovascular Bundle

The lateral pelvic fascia is incised at the apex and midportion of the prostate and a plane is developed between the neurovascular bundle and prostatic fascia. The dissection is continued posteriorly until it meets the plane initially developed between the prostate and rectum. The pedicle is then ligated above the neurovascular bundle.

Antegrade Nerve Sparing

The interfascial plane between the rectum and prostate is developed to the apex of the prostate. The pedicles are then thinned using blunt and sharp dissection proceeding in a medial to lateral direction. The dissection then proceeds anteriorly towards the apex of the prostate.

Summary

Since its introduction in 1999, the da Vinci Surgical System, with its improved ergonomics, wristed instrumentation, and magnified, three-dimensional visualization, has become an integral tool in urologic surgery.

This chapter highlights the technique of robotic prostatectomy and describes techniques to maximize the Trifecta outcomes of cancer control, urinary continence, and erectile function.

With increasing experience, refinements in technique have resulted in improved outcomes for patients. Future areas of research should focus on developing patient-specific surgical protocols based on risk stratification that further enhance quality of life and cure for our patients.

Suggested Reading

1. Beck SM, Skarecky D, Miller S, Ahlering TE. Athermal tension adjustable suture ligation of the vascular pedicle during robot-assisted prostatectomy. J Endourol. 2012;26:834–7.
2. Chauhan S, Coelho RF, Rocco B, Palmer KJ, et al. Techniques of Nerve-Sparing and Potency Outcomes Following Robot-Assisted Laparoscopic Prostatectomy. Int Braz J Urol. 2010;36:259–72.
3. Correa JJ, Pow-Sang JM. Optimizing Cancer Control and Functional Outcomes Following Robotic Prostatectomy. Cancer Control. 2010;17:233–44.
4. Ghani KR, Trinh Q, Menon M. Vattikuti Institute Prostatectomy-Technique. J Endourol. 2012;2012: 1558–65.
5. Turpen R, Atalah H, Su L. Tecchnical Advances in Robot-assisted Laparoscopic Radical Prostatectomy. Ther Adv Urol. 2010;1:251–8.
6. Vora AA, Dajani D, Lynch JH, Kowalczyk KJ. Anatomic and Technical Considerations for Optimizing Recovery of Urinary Function during Robotic-assisted Radical Prostatectomy. Curr Opin Urol. 2013;23:78–87.

Perineal Prostatectomy

7

Nikhil Khattar, Rishi Nayyar, and Rajeev Sood

Introduction

The oncologic world is still searching for the ideal surgical procedure for treatment of localized prostate cancer. This would provide excellent oncological control, acceptable continence, preserve potency when indicated, and be minimally invasive and cost-effective.

The perineal approach for radical prostatectomy was described by HH Young more than a hundred years ago. It remained the preferred approach for radical prostatectomy for many decades before Walsh described anatomical radical retropubic rrostatectomy (RRP) in 1975–1976. The popularity of the perineal approach declined considerably in the next two decades as retropubic approach promised better continence and potency rates because of the possible nerve sparing that it could offer. It was only after the anatomical principles of retropubic approach were applied to the perineal route [1] and the understanding that pelvic lymphadenectomy

could be omitted in selected cases, the perineal approach started gaining popularity again. The only shortcoming that remained was the inability to perform lymphadenectomy. The recent descriptions of feasibility of pelvic lymphadenectomy through the same perineal incision have ushered in a new phase in radical perineal prostatectomy (RPP) and now it is being considered as a truly minimally invasive, cost-effective option even in the era of robotic assisted radical prostatectomy (RARP).

Surgical Anatomy Relevant to Perineal Approach

The anatomical aspects that require in-depth understanding in relation to RPP are (a) anatomy between the prostate and rectum to which not many urologists are familiar, (b) the nomenclature of the fasciae covering the prostate, (c) the anatomy of the puboprostatic complex which explains how the dorsal venous complex (DVC) is saved during the dissection, and (d) the anatomy relevant to nerve preservation.

There are cadaveric studies that have specifically looked into macroscopic and microscopic anatomical details of the perineum and the puboprostatic complex with special reference to perineal approaches for prostatectomy. Fasciae related to the prostate have also been reviewed with special emphasis on correct nomenclature. The neuroanatomy related to the prostate is also

N. Khattar, M.B.B.S., M.S., M.Ch. (Urol.) (✉)
R. Nayyar, M.S., M.Ch., F.M.A.S.
R. Sood, M.B.B.S., M.S. (Surg.)., M.Ch. (Urol.)
Department of Urology, PGIMER and Dr Ram Manohar Lohia Hospital, New Delhi, India
e-mail: drkhattar@gmail.com

R.V. Khanna et al. (eds.), *Surgical Techniques for Prostate Cancer*,
DOI 10.1007/978-1-4939-1616-0_7, © Springer Science+Business Media New York 2015

Fig. 7.1 Depiction of anatomy in the midsagittal plane along with two approaches for RPP. *BL* bladder, *P* prostate, *RH* rhabdosphincter, *RU* rectourethralis; puboprostatic complex consists of puboprostatic ligaments (PPL—*red*); intermediate pubourethral ligament (*yellow*) and anterior pubourethral ligament (PUL—*green*). Note the dorsal vein of penis continuing over prostate as DVC

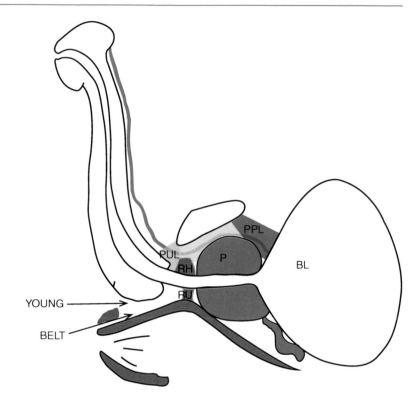

evolving from the classic description of a well-defined neurovascular bundle to a "trizonal concept." The mentioned publications form the basis of the following anatomical description and have been cited at appropriate places. These anatomical details are inseparable from the actual operative steps, but for the sake of proper understanding, they have been described separately.

The Anatomy Between the Prostate and the Rectum

As both halves of the levator ani muscle, after originating from the white line across the pelvic wall, descend down in form of curved curtains to cup the prostate deep in the pelvis, its most medial fibers, the puboanalis, never join each other in the retropubic space (separated by 10–30 mm space) [2] but instead form a sling around the rectum. This sling marks the junction of the rectum with the anal canal. Beyond this point, the anal canal is angulated backwards to culminate at the anal orifice. At the same level lies the prostatomembranous junction. Thus in the midsaggital plane the membranous urethra is surrounded by the Ω-shaped smooth muscle rhabdosphincer which is bulky anteriorly and the rectourethralis posteriorly. The rectourethralis occupies the gap between the right and left portions of the sling of levator ani between the urethra and the rectum. It contains smooth muscle fibers which interdigitate posteriorly with the longitudinal smooth muscle fibers of the rectum [2] and also insert in the perineal body and the bulb of the urethra [3]. The external anal sphincter (consisting of deep, superficial and subcutaneous parts) surrounds the lower third of the anal canal whereas the internal anal sphincter encircles the upper two-thirds. The Young approach to perineal prostatectomy is suprasphincteric and does not damage any anal sphincter whereas the Belt approach is subsphincteric and involves stretching of the anal sphincteric muscles and consequently more chances of anal incontinence (Fig. 7.1).

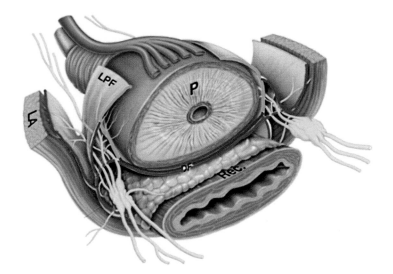

Fig. 7.2 Prostate with its covering fasciae. The levator ani (LA) fascia (*purple*) is the parietal endopelvic fascia which reflects over the prostate as visceral endopelvic fascia to fuse with the lateral prostatic fascia (LPF—*green*). The Denonvillier's fascia (DF) proper (*red*) is located on the posterior aspect of prostate. Another ventral layer of DF is actually the ventral rectal fascia (*blue*). The main bulk of neuronal tissue passes at the confluence of these fascia between the layers. Modified from Costello et al. Immunohistochemical study of the cavernous nerves in the periprostatic region. BJU Int. 2011 Apr;107(8):1210–5. With permission from John Wiley and Sons

Nomenclature of Fasciae Around the Prostate (Fig. 7.2)

The ventral rectal fascia (posterior layer of Denonvillier's fascia): As we go in the space between the anal canal and the bulb of the penis over the surface of external anal sphincter toward the prostate, after division of the rectourethralis muscle, we encounter the prostate covered with a shiny fascia which is the ventral rectal fascia or the fascia propria of the rectum (wrongly called the posterior layer of Denonvillier's fascia) [4]. This fascial layer covers the ventral surface of the rectum and is continuous with the lateral rectal fascia which covers the lateral aspect of rectum. It descends in front of the rectum behind the prostate to fuse with the perineal body. As we cut the rectourethralis by keeping a downward traction over the surface of the anal canal, the space between the prostate and the rectum opens up with the ventral rectal fascia staying over the prostate.

Denonvillier's fascia (anterior layer of Denonvillier's fascia): It is derived from embryonic fusion of the two layers of peritoneum of the prostatorectal cul de sac. These layers are not actually separable. While descending behind the bladder, it loosely covers the seminal vesicles but lower down is densely adherent to the underlying prostate. It usually extends up to the apex of the prostate.

Lateral pelvic fascia: It is the fascia covering the medial surface of the levator ani and is actually the parietal layer of endopelvic fascia [5].

Lateral prostatic fascia: It is the fascia immediately surrounding the prostate especially anteriorly and laterally. Posteriorly it is fused with and is inseparable from Denonvillier's fascia. Some consider this fascia to be a multilayered [4] visceral component of endopelvic fascia. This contains some nerve fibers that form the accessory distal neural pathways (see later) of the cavernous nerves and is preserved in "veil of Aphrodite" technique [6].

Prostatic capsule: There is no true capsule over the prostate. A fibromuscular tissue surrounds the prostate which is indistinct from and is a part of underlying prostatic stroma [5].

Fig. 7.3 With straight Lowsley tractor depressed toward rectum, space can be created on the anterior surface of prostate (*arrow*). With the prostate thus rotated, the DVC automatically remains away from surgical field. Note the anterior pubourethral ligament (*green*) still attached to the urethra keeping it suspended

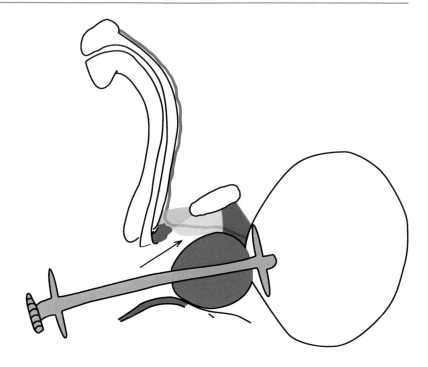

The Anatomy of the Puboprostatic Complex

Puboprostatic complex refers to the structures between the pubic symphysis and the anterior aspect of the prostate and proximal urethra. It is responsible for keeping the prostate and proximal urethra suspended behind the pubic symphysis (Fig. 7.1). Steiner [7] and Wimpissinger et al. [8] independently studied the anatomy of the puboprostatic complex in detail during surgical as well as cadaveric dissections. It consists of **(i) puboprostatic ligaments (or the posterior pubourethral ligaments)**: they are the most proximal pyramidal structures and are said to be lying in a horizontal plane keeping the bladder neck and the proximal prostate suspended to the pubic symphysis, **(ii) the DVC**: it is the continuation of dorsal vein of penis into the retropubic space and runs beneath the pubic arch separated from the anterior surface of prostate by the **(iii) fibromuscular connective tissue (or the intermediate pubourethral ligament)**: this fibromuscular soft tissue connects the anterior commissure of the prostate to the undersurface of the pubic wall. It is oriented in a vertical plane

and together with the puboprostatic ligament, forms a "T"-shaped structure **(iv) the pubourethral ligament proper (or the anterior pubourethral ligament)** which holds the membranous urethra suspended. During the perineal approach, while dissecting at the prostatic apex, when the urethra is transected, the anterior pubourethral ligament is left undisturbed attached with the urethra and we enter the retropubic space. The insertion of the straight Lowsley through the transected apex helps downward rotation of the prostate to bring anterior prostatic surface in view. Here we bluntly separate the intermediate pubourethral ligament and further push the DVC away from the prostatic surface to allow working in an avascular plane (Fig. 7.3).

This step has two major implications, namely, avoidance of DVC, resulting in less blood loss as compared to other approaches, and preservation of urethral suspensory mechanism which helps in achieving good "early continence" rates.

The concept of preservation of the urethral suspensory mechanism for improvement of the continence rates during the retropubic approach was introduced in the early 1990s [9]. However, it was always a natural part of the

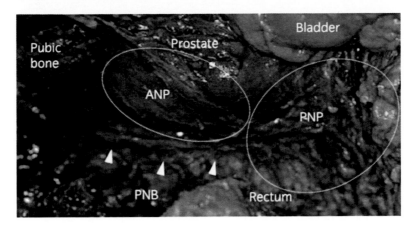

Fig. 7.4 Neuronal structures around prostate as visualized during robotic surgery. The "Trizonal concept" of Taenaka and Tewari. *PNP* proximal neurovascular plate (overlying the rectum), *PNB* predominant neurovascular bundle (posterolaterally), *ANP* accessory distal neural pathways (over the lateral surface). From Takenaka A., Tewari AK. Anatomical basis for carrying out a state-of-the-art radical prostatectomy. International Journal of Urology (2012) 19, 7–19. Reprinted with permission from John Wiley and Sons

perineal approach since it leaves the pubourethral ligament anatomy undisturbed from its attachment on the pubic bone by virtue of dissection on the surface of prostate.

The Anatomy for Nerve Preservation

The neuroanatomy relevant to nerve preservation during radical prostatectomy is still evolving. Even after Walsh and Donker's "discovery" [10] and wide application of the technique of preservation of neurovascular bundles (NVB) in the years that followed, the outcomes of erectile function were variable (56–93 %) [11]. The traditional concept that the cavernous nerves arise from the pelvic splanchnic nerves and autonomic plexus in front of and lateral to the rectum at the level just above the seminal vesicles and travel caudally in "cord-like" NVB on the posterolateral surface of prostate has been modified by recent anatomical studies. Takenaka and Tewari [12], in a review of contemporary anatomical studies, described that the relevant neural tissue encountered during radical prostatectomy rests in three zones (the **"Trizonal"** concept) (Fig. 7.4). The zones are: **(i) proximal neurovascular plate (PNP)**: The neural tissue arising from the pelvic

splanchnic nerves is located in a broad area extending from underneath the seminal vesicles to laterally over the lateral rectal fascia. This plate of tissue carries all the candidate fibers of the cavernous nerves, which cannot be identified surgically, and hence the entire broad plate needs to be preserved at this proximal level. Distally, some fibers converge to form the **(ii) predominant neurovascular bundle (PNB)**, which is the classically described NVB travelling on the posterolateral surface of the prostate. A few other fibers remain divergent over the lateral prostatic fascia as **(iii) accessory distal neural pathways (ANP)** and form an additional conduit for neural transmission. An earlier anatomical study by the same author on 14 formalin fixed male cadavers found that the pelvic splanchnic nerves does not solely carry parasympathetic fibers as earlier thought, but also consists of up to 36 % sympathetic fibers and consequently the nerves in the above-described zones are also contributing to the continence mechanisms in addition to erectile function [13].

NVB preservation alone might be giving variable results as the other two zones are not preserved. Better erectile function claimed in other techniques like high anterior release [14] and "veil of Aphrodite" nerve preservation [15] can be ascribed to respecting these evolving anatomical concepts. Another immunohistochemical study of periprostatic areas on cadavers however contradicts these findings by concluding that between 3 and 9 o'clock there is hardly any significant parasympathetic nerve distribution and that there is no anatomical evidence to practice these higher incisions [16]. A limitation of the study however was that only four cadavers were studied, two fresh and two fixed. The nerve sparing technique in RPP as described by Weldon, although not yet studied as extensively as it has been for other approaches, respects the above anatomical description and is mentioned later.

Indications

Traditionally, RPP has been advocated either when lymphadenectomy could be safely omitted, i.e. low-risk disease where risk of positive nodes would be less than 5 % according to Partin's tables (serum PSA less than 10 ng/ml, up to T2a disease, Gleason 6 or 3+4=7) or when laparoscopic pelvic lymphadenectomy was performed along with RPP. Now that the technique of pelvic lymphadenectomy has been developed, it has the potential to broaden the indications to include almost all patients choosing surgical treatment for localized prostatic cancer.

Some special circumstances where perineal approach is particularly suitable are:

- Morbidly obese men [17]
- Post renal transplant recipients [18, 19]
- Prior mesh repair of inguinal hernia [20]

Inability to put the patient in extended lithotomy position would form the only absolute contraindication to this approach. Performing RPP in very small prostate (<20 g), very large prostate (>100 g), and post radiation salvage situations is challenging but not contraindicated.

Preoperative Preparation

On the day prior to surgery, a thorough bowel preparation is given. Antithrombotic stockings and pneumatic compression stockings should be applied prior to surgery. A second generation cephalosporin is used for antibiotic prophylaxis. Blood typing and cross matching are done to keep blood arranged if needed.

Instruments

A set of curved and straight Lowsley tractor (Fig. 7.5) are the only special instruments needed to perform the prostatectomy proper. However, for performing the lymphadenectomy through the same incision, a self-retaining retractor system such as Omnitract™ with various blades and a headlight is absolutely essential.

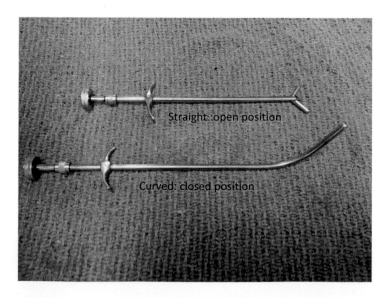

Straight: open position

Curved: closed position

Fig. 7.5 Lowsley tractor

Technique

Position

Patient is positioned in an exaggerated lithotomy position with buttocks protruding from the edge of the table. A rectal shield is placed to facilitate repeated rectal examinations for rectal wall assessment during the surgery to avoid getting in the anal canal or rectum. A curved Lowsley tractor is passed into the bladder and its wings are opened to allow maneuvering the prostate in various stages of dissection. The scrotum is then fixed with sutures so as to prevent falling in front of the perineum.

Approaching the Prostatic Apex

A curved incision is given 2 cm from the anal verge from 9 o'clock to 3 o'clock position remaining medial to the ischial tuberosities. After incising the subcutaneous tissue, bilateral ischiorectal fossae are developed by bluntly entering the index fingers in the visible fat and directing the fingers toward the toes of the operating surgeon (Fig. 7.6a). When in proper space, one should be able to feel the rectum between the two index fingers. Central tendon is then identified and divided (Fig. 7.6b). One can then identify the circular fibers of the anal sphincter (Fig. 7.6c).

Two popular approaches for reaching the apex of the prostate from here are the traditional Young approach (suprasphincteric) and Belt (subsphincteric) approach. With the Belt approach there is more chance of anal sphincteric incontinence [2]. With sharp and blunt dissection in the midline between the anal canal and the bulb of penis, the fibers of rectourethralis are identified and sharply divided transversely not deviating from the midline (Fig. 7.7a). The direction of this dissection is not parallel to the floor but slightly upward toward the apex of the prostate which can be identified by gently shaking the Lowsley toward and away from the abdomen. Once the apex is identified,

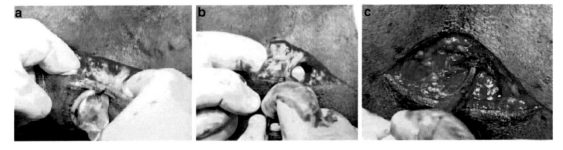

Fig. 7.6 (a) Developing bilateral ischiorectal fossae. (b) Division of the central tendon. (c) Artery forceps passed beneath the circular fibers of external anal sphincter (superficial part)

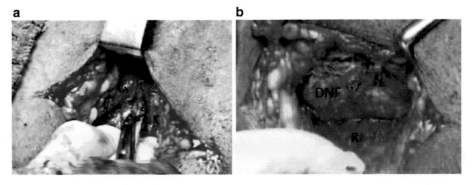

Fig. 7.7 (a) Division of the rectourethralis (note the slightly upward direction of the scissors). (b) Denonvillier's fascia (DNF) over the prostate. *LA* levator ani, *R* rectum

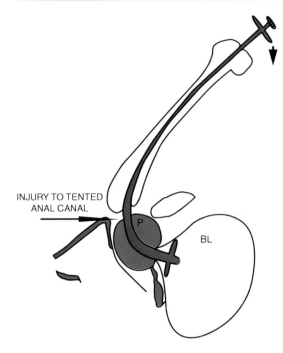

INJURY TO TENTED
ANAL CANAL

P

BL

Fig. 7.8 Assistant's downward traction over the curved Lowsley (towards abdomen) in order to bring the prostate towards the incision for better view during apical dissection leads to a tented anal canal and makes it more prone to injury.

the rectum can be swept in caudad direction with the help of Kittner dissector to expose the shiny Denonvillier's fascia of the prostate (Fig. 7.7b).

One of the common modes for the rectum to get injured is when the assistant depresses the curved Lowsley tractor in order to bring the prostate toward the wound, thereby tenting the rectum further (Fig. 7.8). A useful modification to the technique of exposing the prostate is the delayed introduction of curved Lowsley after the recto-urethralis is divided [21]. This prevents any distortion of the anatomy at this stage as the rectum most commonly gets injured before the prostate is exposed [3].

Mobilization of the Lateral Surfaces and Base of Prostate

Laterally on either side the prostate is closely invested by levator ani muscles. Space can be created by inserting the finger bluntly between the prostate and the levator muscle (Fig. 7.9). This is facilitated by turning the curved Lowsley tractor to the side of the lateral surface being freed in order to push the prostate to the opposite side to open up this space.

The assistant is then asked to hold the Lowsley inferiorly toward the surgeon so that the prostate is held in a "hung up" position (Jewett maneuver) which facilitates development of space between the base of the prostate and seminal vesicles, covered with Denonvillier's fascia, and the rectum. Constant caudad traction over the rectum with a thin Deaver is required and using either two Kittner dissectors or a gauze piece wrapped over a suction tip pushed slowly between the rectum and the prostate, a space is developed [20]. While doing this the lateral prostatic pedicles that come into view can be put to stretch by moving the Lowsley tractor to either side and can be ligated or clipped and divided. Having cleared the pedicles, one can feel the open blades of the Lowsley tractor at the bladder neck laterally and the vesicoprostatic junction can be defined all around except anteriorly.

Dissecting Seminal Vesicles

Traditionally this step was performed after transection of the bladder neck but all contemporary techniques emphasize on dissecting out seminal vesicles prior to opening the bladder if possible. This preference has developed after it was theorized that incomplete removal of Seminal Vesicles (SVs) during RPP is responsible for higher incidence of early biochemical recurrence (BCR) [22]. After development of space between the rectum and prostate and beyond the base of prostate, the Denonvillier's fascia overlying the SVs is incised transversely exposing the SV and vas deferens. With the help of a Mixter forceps, each vas is hooked out, clipped, and divided as proximally as possible followed by dissection and delivery of the seminal vesicles one by one after dealing with the seminal vesicular artery at the tip of each SV [23].

Fig. 7.9 Finger dissection between prostate (P) and levator ani (LA) creates a space between them

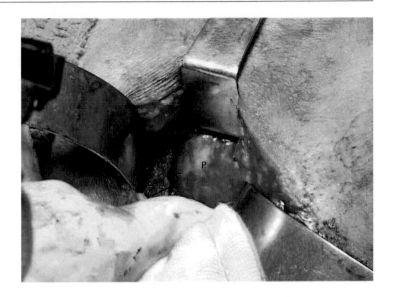

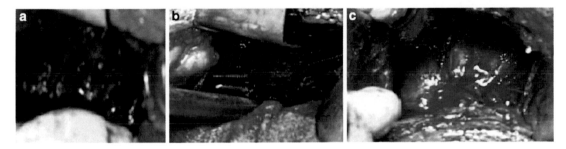

Fig. 7.10 (**a**) At prostatic apex, with the posterior wall of urethra divided, Lowsley can be seen shining. (**b**) Anterior wall of urethra ready to be divided. (**c**) Downward depression on straight Lowsley tractor brings anterior surface in view. *PPL* puboprostatic ligaments

Dissection of Apex and Intraprostatic Urethral Dissection

At the apex, the urethra can be palpated over the Lowsley tractor where it exits the prostate. It can be encircled with a right angled forceps in this area. While doing this, the dorsal vein is automatically pushed dorsally away from urethra. The prostate often, especially if large, overhangs the membranous urethra by a few millimeters at the apex. Dissection within this overhanging prostate is required in such cases to get to the true prostatomembranous junction before its division. This is easily accomplished by gentle use of a right angled forceps to dig out the true prostatomembranous junction. The importance of preserving the urethral length proximal to rhabdo-sphincter was always insisted but recently it has been seen that it can safely be preserved up to verumontanum without compromising the onco-logical outcome and this helps in significant improvement of early continence at 3 months [24].

Transection of the Urethra and Anterior Dissection

At the prostato-urethral junction, the posterior wall of urethra is divided transversely with a no. 15 blade and after the curved Lowsley is clearly visible (Fig. 7.10a) it is replaced with a straight Lowsley passed in the bladder directly

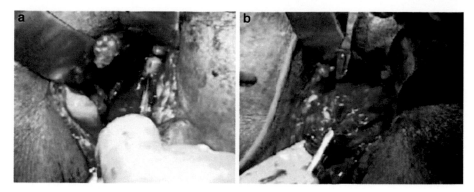

Fig. 7.11 (**a**) Anterior bladder wall is opened over wing of straight Lowsley felt at bladder neck. (**b**) Division of the posterior bladder wall after confirming that the orifices are away

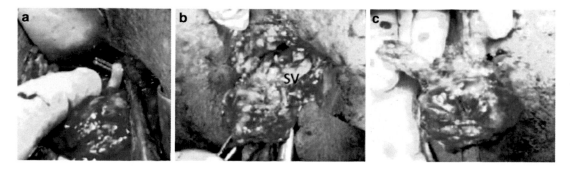

Fig. 7.12 (**a**) The vas deferens brought out over a right angled forceps. (**b**) Seminal vesicle (SV) with some pedicular tissue still attached. (It is preferable to dissect SVs prior to opening of the bladder.) (**c**) The complete specimen after an extrafascial dissection

through the operative area. The anterior wall of the urethra is then divided similarly over the right angled forceps (Fig. 7.10b). Sutures may be taken in the anterior urethral wall at this time, when it is visible, for subsequent anastomosis. Keeping a downward traction on the straight Lowsley tractor, the anterior surface of the prostate is then bluntly dissected. The puboprostatic ligaments can be identified at this stage (Fig. 7.10c) and they are sharply divided no farther than the level of bladder neck. The DVC gets pushed automatically and does not come into the picture (see Fig. 7.3).

Defining Bladder Neck and Transection

The above step exposes the anterior bladder neck which can be confirmed by rotating the straight Lowsley to feel its wing through the anterior bladder wall at the bladder neck (Fig. 7.11a). The bladder is opened at this point and the straight Lowsley is then replaced with either a Foley catheter or a penrose drain which enters the prostatic urethra and comes out through this opening to loop and maneuver the prostate during further dissection. A curved scissors is used to transect the anterior bladder neck. A thin Deaver retractor is passed in the bladder through this opening and used to retract the bladder wall to help identify the ureteric orifices before one sharply divides the posterior wall of the bladder (Fig. 7.11b). The Deaver retractor is then shifted to a subtrigonal position in the plane between bladder and seminal vesicles. If not already dissected, the vas and SVs are then dissected and the SV arteries are clipped on either side to deliver the specimen (Fig. 7.12). The rectum is inspected for any inadvertent injury before the anastomosis.

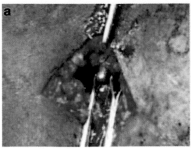 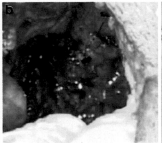 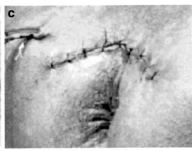

Fig. 7.13 (**a**) The urethra (with metal dilator protruding out) and the bladder edges (held in Babcock forceps) are usually right in front and close to each other making vesi-courethral anastomosis easier. (**b**) Completed anastomosis. (**c**) Sutured incision line with a tube drain coming out separately

Vesicourethral Anastomosis

Before the anastomosis, if the bladder opening is wide, the bladder is sutured to itself starting from 6 o'clock till the size of the bladder opening is approximately 30 Fr. This "racquet handle" closure also secures the ureteric orifices in a position away from vesicourethral anastomosis. A 2-0 Monocryl® (poliglecaprone 25) suture on a 5/8 circle needle is used for the anastomosis. Six interrupted stitches over a 3 way 18 Fr catheter are enough for a secure anastomosis. As both the urethral end and the bladder are right in front at the level of the eyes, the anastomosis is relatively easier to perform than in other techniques of radical prostatectomy (Fig. 7.13). A gloved drain or a closed suction drain is placed close to but not directly behind the anastomotic line. Before closure, the fibers of the rectourethralis are sutured to the bulb of the penis and the central tendon is reapproximated. Skin is then closed with nylon sutures or staples.

Technique of Nerve Sparing

Weldon and Tavel [1] are credited for the description of nerve sparing technique in RPP. Nerve sparing is indicated in men who have good preoperative erectile function and have either T1 disease (bilateral nerve sparing) or T2a disease (unilateral nerve sparing). After mobilization of the lateral surface and base of the prostate, a longitudinal midline incision is given on the ventral rectal fascia on the surface of prostate (posterior layer of Denonvillier's fascia). The incision can be extended on either side toward the base in an inverted Y fashion if a bilateral nerve sparing is planned. The fascia along with the NVB (the PNB) is lifted away from prostatic surface along the entire length of this incision. Any attachments to the prostatic surface are clipped avoiding electrocautery use. The NVB is mobilized distally up to 1 cm beyond the prostatourethral junction and proximally up to the prostatic base. This allows moving the entire fascial layer laterally (including PNB and ANP) so that it does not get stretched during maneuvering of the prostate. The levator ani is left covered with these fascial layers in a nerve sparing dissection whereas in a non-nerve sparing dissection, the fibers lie bare (Fig. 7.14). If there is induration preventing the release of this fascial layer, ipsilateral nerve excision is performed.

Technique of Perineal Pelvic Lymphadenectomy

Inability to sample pelvic lymph nodes has been a major handicap of RPP. Consequently the indications were limited to a select group of patients with low risk of positive lymph nodes if simultaneous laparoscopic pelvic lymphadenectomy was not being planned. To circumvent this shortcoming and to provide wider applicability of the procedure, surgeons from Japan and Germany have performed pioneering work by introducing

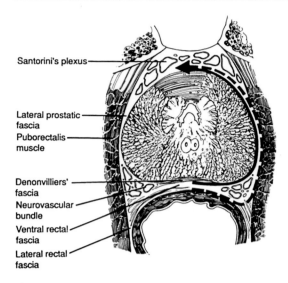

Santorini's plexus

Lateral prostatic fascia

Puborectalis muscle

Denonvilliers' fascia

Neurovascular bundle

Ventral rectal fascia

Lateral rectal fascia

Fig. 7.14 In non-nerve sparing dissection (*dotted line*), the ventral rectal fascia, the neurovascular bundle, and the lateral prostatic fascia are included in the specimen baring the levator ani fibers. In nerve sparing dissection (*continuous line*) after incising the ventral rectal fascia in midline, the fascial layer including the neurovascular bundle, is lifted off the prostate. From Weldon, V. E.: Technique of modern radical perineal prostatectomy. Urology,60:689, 2002. Reprinted with permission from Elsevier Limited

pelvic lymphadenectomy through the same perineal incision. Saito and Murakami [25, 26] started performing removal of obturator and internal iliac lymph nodes along with partial external iliac lymphadenectomy through perineal incision. The yield of lymph nodes was an average of eight nodes in 20 patients. This could not be considered reliable in high-risk patients. Keller et al. modified the technique and performed extended lymph node dissection in 90 consecutive patients up to the level of crossing of ureter with average of 19 nodes removed with no major complications [27] (Fig. 7.15).

The lymphadenectomy is performed after the prostate is removed. The endopelvic fascia is pierced and the perivesical space is entered. The bladder is pushed medially and is retained there with the help of self-retaining system. The space can also be created with the help of a trocar mounted balloon device. The obturator nerve is the first to get identified followed by external iliac vessels in the order of depth. Keeping a slight pull at the lymphatic tissue with an Allis clamp, the nodes are gradually teased away from

the vessels going deeper till the ureter can be identified. Hemoclips are used for the lymphatic vessels. A silicon drain is kept at the nodal dissection site on each side for a few days till the secretions are minimal.

Other Modifications and Their Usefulness

Endoscope Assisted RPP

As bladder neck is the most poorly visualized part during perineal approach especially in larger glands, it has been described to incise the bladder neck all around at the prostatovesical junction with the help of Collin's knife [28]. The resectoscope is inserted through the transected prostatic apex during RPP. The endoscopic assistance has not been used by most of the perineal surgeons; however, it may be useful in cases of post TURP prostates [29].

Extended RPP (Removal of DVC Along with Prostate)

The bladder neck anteriorly is the most common site for a positive surgical margin (PSM) following RPP as that is the farthest and most poorly visualized area during the operation in contrast to retropubic approaches where apex is the most favored site. To reduce this risk and to bring it technically even more close to retropubic approach, extended RPP has been described where the DVC is divided with harmonic scalpel [30]. Extended RPP has the potential to decrease the rates of anterior PSMs.

The Management During Postoperative Phase

Postoperatively all patients are allowed liquid diet on the evening of surgery and semisolids from next day onward. Patient is allowed ambulation from the first postoperative day. Need for parenteral analgesia does not exceed more than 2 days followed by on demand oral analgesics. Perineal drain output usually remains minimal

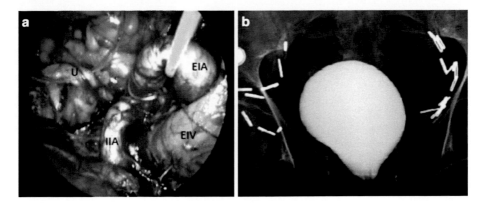

Fig. 7.15 (**a**) Left perivesical space after completed lymphadenectomy through perineal route (shown with the help of laparoscopic camera). *EIA* external iliac artery, *EIV* external iliac vein, *IIA* internal iliac artery, *U* ureter (looped at the level of crossing of iliac vessels). (**b**) Postoperative X-ray with metal clips depicting the extent of lymphadenectomy that is possible. From Keller H, Lehmann J, Beier J. Radical Perineal Prostatectomy and Simultaneous Extended Pelvic Lymph Node Dissection via the Same Incision. Eur. Urol.; 52 (2007) 384–388. Reprinted with permission from Elsevier

and is removed within 48 h of surgery. Patient can be discharged with urethral catheter after drain removal. Catheter removal is done in the office setting between 7 and 10 days.

Results

In a recent review of literature, Wronsky compared results of RPP with all other techniques including RARP [31]. His chart (Table 7.1) compares all issues relevant to the outcome of RPP, including intraoperative and postoperative complications, oncologic outcome parameters (PSM and BCR), functional outcome parameters (Erectile dysfunction (ED) and continence), and cost with other techniques. A glance at this table justifies their questioning of RARP as the "gold standard." The review concludes by quoting Laurent Boccon-Gibod from an editorial in *European Urology*: "There is no doubt that as far as pain, complications, transfusion rate, continence, positive margins, and cosmesis, RPP meets every goal of a minimally invasive surgery [32]."

Oncological Outcome (PSM and BCR)

In a study to look for predictors of PSM after RPP, clinical T stage and biopsy Gleason sum were not found to be predictors for PSM whereas smaller prostate volume was found to be correlating with higher chances of PSM [33].

The location of PSM is more commonly toward the apex in all retropubic approaches and toward the anterior surface and bladder neck in the perineal approach. This difference is because the region most difficult to access in retropubic approaches is the apex whereas in RPP the apex is well visualized and instead the bladder neck is farthest and poorly visualized. The anterior surface becomes a favored location because the capsule is exposed there as DVC is not included in the specimen [3]. A positive margin, incomplete removal of seminal vesicle [3, 21], and capsular incisions [34] are associated with increased biochemical failure rates. In contrast an SV sparing RPP has also been described with equivalent oncological outcomes [35].

Table 7.1 Prostatectomy approaches in outline

Contributory factor	Perineal prostatectomy	Retropubic prostatectomy	Laparoscopic prostatectomy	RARP
Indications and patient selections	Not limited in every respect	Previous abdominal surgery or unfavorable body habitus are the main constraints		
Invasiveness	Minimal	Contemporary not very extensive	Minimal	Minimal
Concurrent lymphadenectomy	Technically demanding, only as staging procedure	Without limits as curative and/or staging procedure		
Average time of procedure	The shortest 35–120 min	110–197 min	Comparable 170–270 min	141–160 min
Transfusion rate	Low and comparable, up to 3 %			
Intraoperative rectal laceration	The highest rate among approaches 1–11 %	Comparable and less than 10 %. Rectal fistulas develop in 1.5–3.6 % of patients		
Wound infection	Approximately 5 %	Approximately 5–9 %	Approximately 1 %	
Length of catheterization	Mostly 7–14 days regardless of approach			
Avg. hospitalization (days, in Europe)	7.9	Considerable differences between centers	6.8	4.3
Perioperative mortality rate	Comparable and low, ranging 0.3–1 %			
Positive surgical margins rate	16.3–24.7 %	12–25 %	11–30 %	Up to 27.3 %
SM+ sites specific for approach	25 % anterior, 16 % posterolateral	48–58 % apex, 19–40 % posterior aspect, 19 % prostate base	50 % apical, 30 % posterolateral, 20 % prostate base	50 % apical and posterolateral site
Postoperative risk of anastomotic stricture	1–3.8 %	5.5 %	0.6–4.1 %	Up to 4 %
Late oncological outcomes PSA recurrence	Equivalent in organ-confined, specimen-confined, and SM+ groups of patients for all prostatectomy techniques			
Continence return 1 year after surgery	81–96 %	61–97.1 %	80.7–91.9 %	86.3–91.8 %
Return of potency for nerve sparing procedures	Depends on definition of postoperative potency (no uniform and unambiguous criteria for classification)			
	41–80 %	50–55 %	52.5–65 %	53–81 %
Patient's satisfaction with chosen treatment	Up to 95 %	87.1–89.2 %	Up to 98 %	80.1 % (the highest rate of disappointment)
Approximate costs of procedure per case	Less than $5,000	Fundamental differences between countries, health-care systems, and centers. The following financial reports from Texas Southwestern Medical Center		
		$3,989–5,141	$4,941–5,905	$6,283–7,369
		+$185	+$725	+$2,015
		+$1,611	+$2,453	+$2,798
				+$2,698
Charges for cash payers (USA)	$11,600	$34,000	Not reported	$42,000
Learning curve (as compared with RRP)	Longer	Frame of reference	Longer	Longer (but shorter than laparoscopic)

Synopsis of article issues

From Wroński S. Radical perineal prostatectomy—the contemporary resurgence of a genuinely minimally invasive procedure: Procedure outline. Comparison of the advantages, disadvantages, and outcomes of different surgical techniques of treating organ-confined prostate cancer (PCa). A literature review with special focus on perineal prostatectomy Cent European J Urol. 2012; 65(4): 188–194. Copyright Polish Urological Association. Open Access

Functional Outcome: Continence and Erectile Dysfunction

Although the attempts to compare the erectile function and continence outcomes between different techniques are marred because of lack of standard definition of both potency and continence, the results are still comparable. A younger age and a good preoperative erectile function are associated with better preservation of erectile function after nerve sparing surgery. Albayrak and colleagues specifically studied the early continence outcomes after RPP in 120 patients and reported that more than a third were immediately continent as soon as the catheter was removed and at 3 months 72.5 % were continent, i.e., "early continence" [36]. These early continence results are exceptionally encouraging. Overall, the results are comparable or even better than other approaches for radical prostatectomy.

Practice of nerve sparing techniques in RPP is relatively new and was described by Weldon and Tavel. In Weldon's own experience, an unassisted potency rate after nerve sparing in RPP in selected men approached 70 % [22]. In Harris' experience 67 of 84 bilaterally nerve spared patients recovered partial erections at 24 months [37]. Brehmer et al. reported 48 % recovery of unassisted intercourse in 31 patients with more than 2 years follow-up after unilateral nerve sparing [38]. In all retropubic routes, once the NVBs or plates are dissected away, the prostate is lifted off them without causing any further stretching. Whereas in RPP, even after dissecting away the fascia containing the neurovascular tissue, it is subjected to a lot of manipulation and stretching while trying to deliver the gland thereby increasing the risk of laceration of neurovascular tissue [39]. Not many studies have reported on nerve sparing, and literature on results is yet to evolve.

Complications

Rectal Injury

Although the incidence of rectal injury is high, when it is intraoperatively identified and sutured in 2 layers, it does not result in further consequences. Only 3 of 22 patients with rectal lacerations during 451 RPPs required colostomy for their management [40]. In a relatively recent Brazilian experience of 176 patients, authors report a low incidence of rectal lacerations and rectal fistulas (5.7 % and 2.3 % respectively) [41]. Apart from the natural risk that the perineal approach poses to the anorectal integrity, it is the relatively smaller number of cases in each series as compared to RRP or RARP that explains the higher incidence.

Fecal Incontinence

In 1998 Bishoff et al. reported a startling incidence of fecal incontinence in 18 % of their RPP patients as compared to 5 % of RRP patients and started off this debate [42]. The method of their data collection was a telephonic survey after at least 1 year from the date of surgery. There was no baseline to compare with. Steineck et al. [43] in 2002 studied the quality of life in 376 men, randomized to either radical prostatectomy or watchful waiting, at least 12 months after surgery (RRP in all cases) and 14 months after randomization. Seven percent of RRP patients and 10 % of watchful waiting patients had some kind of fecal soiling. The fecal incontinence was more than once a week in 1 % and 6 % patients, respectively. They concluded that radical prostatectomy does not lead to de novo fecal incontinence and the previous reports were because of lack of a control group and a baseline evaluation. Korman and colleagues [44] evaluated bowel function in 150 consecutive radical prostatectomy patients by a single surgeon (79 RPP, 71 RRP). They also had a control group of 75 prostatic biopsy patients. At 1 year the fecal incontinence rates were 5.4, 6.4, and 4.8 %, respectively, for RPP, RRP, and control groups. A group from Turkey manometrically assessed the anorectal complications after both the approaches and found that although both external and internal anal sphincteric pressures decrease significantly after RPP as compared to RRP, clinically there is no difference (anal incontinence scores were not significantly different) [45].

Anastomotic Stricture

Harris reported anastomotic stricture in only 1 % of his single surgeon series of 704 cases [36]. In a large single center comparison of 866 RPPs and 2,052 RRPs, Gillitzer et al. reported incidence of anastomotic strictures to be 3.8 % and 5.5 %, respectively [46]. As the vesicourethral anastomosis is performed with relative ease in RPP, the rates of anastomotic strictures are very low as compared to all other techniques including robotic.

Learning RPP

Learning curve for RPP is not as steep as for other minimally invasive radical prostatectomies (MIRP). Many researchers have reported their first experiences with RPP with encouraging results. In a self-appraisal of their first 47 patients that Wrońskiet al. reported [47], 26 patients responded to a questionnaire at least 1 year after surgery. Only 38 % respondents reported some leakage and that too for most of them was only sporadic. Only one patient had continuous urinary leak. We ourselves have reported our initial experience of 35 cases with encouraging results (the incidence of PSMs was 14 % in our series. Continence rates at 3 months and 18 months were 70 % and 92.4 %, respectively, with continence defined as "no pads used") [48].

To evaluate the learning curve for RPP, Fadi Eliya et al., after a 2 day training in RPP, performed RPP in 96 consecutive cases and to determine their learning curve they divided them in 4 almost equal groups according to time period. The perioperative results did not improve significantly from 2nd group onward and they estimated the learning curve for RPP to be approximately 35–40 cases [49].

The Future of RPP

Even after a number of contemporary publications and reviews concluding that RPP is the most cost-effective minimally invasive technique for radical prostatectomy with outcomes equivalent to any other technique including RARP, it is unfortunate that RPP is being performed only by a handful of urologists and is unable to hold its ground firmly. Whether it is the zeal for technology or the pressure of the industry that has become the reason cannot be said conclusively.

Prasad et al. retrospectively reviewed data of more than 9,000 men who underwent radical prostatectomy (RPP, RRP, and MIRP) using SEER (Surveillance, epidemiology and end results)—Medicare linked database in the United States. They observed that the increasing use of MIRP (mainly robotic) had led to "cannibalization" of RPP and RRP. MIRP use was more prevalent in better educated, higher socioeconomic status and those coming from metropolitan cities probably due to effective "marketing." This happened even though MIRP outcomes were not significantly different from those of RRP and RPP resulting in huge cost burdens [50]. Is the market driving the choices?

The realization that an effective tool is being abandoned prematurely is showing up [38, 49, 51]. When it came to effectively handling the growing healthcare burden of prostatic carcinoma in native Africans, RPP was chosen to be taught to African surgeons [52], a step that clearly emphasizes the role it can still play. Well-designed clinical trials are needed to study RPP vs. RARP to prevent denying RPP of whatever potential it has in present era of mounting burden of prostatic cancer. With the constraints of inability to perform lymphadenectomy now removed, RPP has all the potential to become a gold standard for prostate cancer surgery if it is kept alive by "perineourologists."

References

1. Weldon VE, Tavel FR. Potency-sparing radical perineal prostatectomy: anatomy, surgical technique and initial results. J Urol. 1988;140(3):559–62.
2. Matsubara A, Murakami G, Arakawa T, et al. Topographic anatomy of the male perineal structures with special reference to perineal approaches for radical prostatectomy. Int Urol. 2003;10:141–8.
3. Janoff DM, Parra RO. Contemporary appraisal of radical perineal prostatectomy. J Urol. 2005;173: 1863–70.

4. Walz J, Graefen M, Huland H. Basic principles of anatomy for optimal surgical treatment of prostate cancer. World J Urol. 2007;25:31–8.

5. Raychaudhuri B, Cahill D. Pelvic fasciae in urology. Ann R Coll Surg Engl. 2008;90(8):633–7.

6. Mandhani A. Prostatic fascia and recovery of sexual function after radical prostatectomy: is it a "Veil of Aphrodite" or "Veil of mystery"! Indian J Urol. 2009; 25(1):146–8.

7. Steiner MS. The puboprostatic ligament and the male urethral suspensory mechanism: an anatomic study. Urology. 1994;44:530–4.

8. Wimpissinger TF, Tschabitscher M, Feichtinger H, Stackl W. Surgical anatomy of the puboprostatic complex with special reference to radical perineal prostatectomy. BJU Int. 2003;92(7):681–4.

9. Walsh PC, Quinlan DM, Morton RA, Steiner MS. Radical retropubic prostatectomy. Improved anastomosis and urinary continence. Urol Clin North Am. 1990;17(3):679–84.

10. Walsh PC, Donker PJ. Impotence following radical prostatectomy: insight into etiology and prevention. J Urol. 1982;128(3):492–7.

11. Schaeffer EM, Loeb S, Walsh PC. The case for open radical prostatectomy. Urol Clin North Am. 2010; 37(1):49–55.

12. Takenaka A, Tewari AK. Anatomical basis for carrying out a state-of-the-art radical prostatectomy. Int J Urol. 2012;19:7–19.

13. Takenaka A, Kawada M, Murakami G, Hisasue S, Tsukamoto T, Fujisawa M. Intcrindividual variation in distribution of extramural ganglion cells in the male pelves: a semi-quantitative and immunohistochemical study concerning nerve-sparing pelvic surgery. Eur Urol. 2005;48:46–52.

14. Nielsen ME, Schaeffer EM, Marschke P, Walsh PC. High anterior release of the levator fascia improves sexual function following open radical retropubic prostatectomy. J Urol. 2008;180(6):2557–64.

15. Kaul S, Savera A, Badani K, Fumo M, Bhandari A, Menon M. Functional outcomes and oncological efficacy of Vattikuti Institute prostatectomy with Veil of Aphrodite nerve-sparing: an analysis of 154 consecutive patients. BJU Int. 2006;97(3):467–72.

16. Costello AJ, Dowdle BW, Namdarian B, Pedersen J, Murphy DG. Immunohistochemical study of the cavernous nerves in the periprostatic region. BJU Int. 2011;107(8):1210–5.

17. Leung AC, Melman A. Radical perineal prostatectomy: a more optimal treatment approach than laparoscopic radical prostatectomy in obese patients? Rev Urol. 2005;7(1):48–52.

18. Hafron J, Fogarty JD, Wiesen A, Melman A. Surgery for localized prostate cancer after renal transplantation. BJU Int. 2005;95(3):319–22.

19. Yiou R, Salomon L, Colombel M, Patard JJ, Chopin D, Abbou CC. Perineal approach to radical prostatectomy in kidney transplant recipients with localized prostate cancer. Urology. 1999;53(4):822–4.

20. Borchers H, Brehmer B, van Poppel H, Jakse G. Radical prostatectomy in patients with previous groin hernia repair using synthetic nonabsorbable mesh. Urol Int. 2001;67(3):213–5.

21. Melman A, Boczko J, Figueroa J, Leung AC. Critical surgical techniques for radical perineal prostatectomy. J Urol. 2004;171:786–90.

22. Theodorescu D, Lippert MC, Broder SR, Boyd JC. Early prostate-specific antigen failure following radical perineal versus retropubic prostatectomy: the importance of seminal vesicle excision. Urology. 1998;51:277.

23. Weldon VE. Technique of modern radical perineal prostatectomy. Urology. 2002;60:689.

24. Sfoungaristos S, Kontogiannis S, Perimenis P. Early continence recovery after preservation of maximal urethral length until the level of verumontanum during radical prostatectomy: primary oncological and functional outcomes after 1 year of follow-up. Biomed Res Int. 2013;2013:426208. Epub 2013 Sep 19.

25. Saito S, Murakami G. Anatomical study of perineal pelvic lymphadenectomy. Int J Urol. 2007;14: 978–80.

26. Saito S, Murakami G. Radical perineal prostatectomy: novel approach for lymphadenectomy from a perineal incision. J Urol. 2003;170:1298–300.

27. Keller H, Lehmann J, Beier J. Radical perineal prostatectomy and simultaneous extended pelvic lymph node dissection via the same incision. Eur Urol. 2007;52:384–8.

28. Ellison LM, Pinto PA, Kavoussi LR. Radical endoscopic assisted perineal prostatectomy. J Urol. 2003; 170:170–3.

29. Albayrak S, Canguven O, Aydemir H, Goktas C, Cetinel C, Akca O. Endoscope-assisted radical perineal prostatectomy. J Endourol. 2010;24(4):527–30.

30. Inoue S, Shiina H, Sumura M, Urakami S, Matsubara A, Igawa M. Impact of a novel, extended approach of perineal radical prostatectomy on surgical margins in localized prostate cancer. BJU Int. 2010;106:44–8.

31. Wronski S. Radical perineal prostatectomy—the contemporary resurgence of a genuinely minimally invasive procedure: Procedure outline. Comparison of the advantages, disadvantages, and outcomes of different surgical techniques of treating organ-confined prostate cancer (PCa). A literature review with special focus on perineal prostatectomy. Cent European J Urol. 2012;65(4):188–94.

32. Boccon-Gibod L. Radical prostatectomy: open? Laparoscopic? Robotic? Eur Urol. April;49(4): 598–9.

33. Goetzl MA, Krebill R, Griebling TL, Thrasher JB. Predictors of positive surgical margins after radical perineal prostatectomy. Can J Urol. 2009;16(2): 4553–7.

34. Kwak KW, Lee HM, Choi HY. Impact of capsular incision on biochemical recurrence after radical perineal prostatectomy. Prostate Cancer Prostatic Dis. 2010;13(1):28–33.

35. Schäfers S, de Geeter P, Löhmer H, Albers P. Seminal vesicle sparing radical perineal prostatectomy. Urologe A. 2009;48(4):408–14.

36. Albayrak S, Canguven O, Goktas C, Cetinel C, Horuz R, Aydemir H. Radical perineal prostatectomy and early continence: outcomes after 120 cases. Int Braz J Urol. 2010;36(6):693–9.

37. Harris MJ. The anatomic radical perineal prostatectomy: an outcomes-based evolution. Eur Urol. 2007; 52(1):81–8.

38. Brehmer B, Kirschner-Hermanns R, Donner A, Reineke T, Knüchel-Clarke R, Jakse G. Efficacy of unilateral nerve sparing in radical perineal prostatectomy. Urol Int. 2005;74(4):308–14.

39. Comploj E, Pycha A. Experience with radical perineal prostatectomy in the treatment of localized prostate cancer. Ther Adv Urol. 2012;4(3): 125–31.

40. Fichtner J, Gillitzer R, Melchior SW, Hohenfellner M, Thüroff JW. Perineal complications following radical perineal prostatectomy. Aktuelle Urol. 2003;34(4): 223–5.

41. de Arruda HO, Cury J, Ortiz V, Srougi M. Rectal injury in radical perineal prostatectomy. Tumori. 2007;93(6):532–5.

42. Bishoff JT, Motley G, Optenberg SA, Stein CR, Moon KA, Browning SM, Sabanegh E, Foley JP, Thompson IM. Incidence of fecal and urinary incontinence following radical perineal and retropubic prostatectomy in a national population. J Urol. 1998;160(2): 454–8.

43. Steineck G, Helgesen F, Adolfsson J, Dickman PW, Johansson JE, Norlén BJ, Holmberg L. Quality of life after radical prostatectomy or watchful waiting; Scandinavian Prostatic Cancer Group Study Number 4. N Engl J Med. 2002;347(11):790–6.

44. Korman HJ, Mulholland TL, Huang R. Preservation of fecal continence and bowel function after radical perineal and retropubic prostatectomy: a questionnaire-based outcomes study. Prostate Cancer Prostatic Dis. 2004;7(3):249–52.

45. Aydemir H, Albayrak S, Canguven O, Horuz R, Goktas C, Cetinel C, Giral A. Anorectal functions after perineal and retropubic radical prostatectomy—a prospective clinical and anal manometric assessment. Arch Med Sci. 2011;7(1):138–42.

46. Gillitzer R, Thomas C, Wiesner C, Jones J, Schmidt F, Hampel C, Brenner W, Thüroff JW, Melchior SW. Single center comparison of anastomotic strictures after radical perineal and radical retropubic prostatectomy. Urology. 2010;76(2):417–22.

47. Wronski S, Slupski P, Wisniewski P. A single institution study on patient's self-reporting appraisal and functional outcomes of the first set of men following radical perineal prostatectomy. Cent European J Urol. 2012;65(3):124–9.

48. Sood R, Khattar N, Nayyar R, Kathuria S, Narang V, Kaushal D. Case for resurgence of radical perineal prostatectomy in Indian subcontinent. Indian J Urol. 2012;28(4):418–23.

49. Eliya F, Kernen K, Gonzalez J, Peters K, Ibrahim I, Petzel K. Radical perineal prostatectomy: a learning curve? Int Urol Nephrol. 2011;43:139–42.

50. Prasad SM, Gu X, Lavelle R, Lipsitz SR, Hu JC. Comparative effectiveness of perineal versus retropubic and minimally invasive radical prostatectomy. J Urol. 2011;185(1):111–5.

51. Nargund VH, Zaman F. Radical prostatectomy—too soon to abandon the perineal approach? Nat Rev Urol. 2011;8(4):179–80.

52. Ruenes Jr A, Gueye SM. Teaching radical prostatectomy in sub-Saharan Africa. Can J Urol. 2008;15(1):3886–9.

Brachytherapy

8

Matthew C. Ward, Jay P. Ciezki,
and Kevin L. Stephans

Introduction

Prostate brachytherapy offers a convenient and cost-effective treatment option for patients with clinically localized prostate cancer. This minimally invasive technique carries a comparatively low risk of incontinence and impotence [1] while simultaneously avoiding the wider distribution of radiation dose to normal tissue and extended treatment course of conventional external beam radiation.

The implantation of radioactive sources, termed brachytherapy, is one of the earliest forms of radiotherapy. In 1898, only 3 years after Wilhelm Röntgen described the Röntgen Ray, Marie Curie discovered radium, the first known radioactive nucleotide [2, 3]. By 1911, the French physician Octave Pasteau reported the therapeutic effects of radium when used against carcinoma of the prostate, which at that time was considered a rare disease [4]. Hugh Hampton Young, the Johns Hopkins urologist and pioneer of the prostatectomy, revised the implantation of radium needles through 1917 [5]. This was a

primitive procedure by today's standards and was performed without image guidance. With haphazard seed implantation, frequently involving the bladder or rectal wall, nearly every patient experienced significant toxicity and brachytherapy fell out of favor. In 1952, as the limitations of therapeutic castration were realized, the interest in brachytherapy was revitalized by Dr. Rubin Flocks at the University of Iowa [6]. Using an aqueous solution of ^{198}Gold, Dr. Flocks was able to show efficacy in otherwise unresectable cases. Between 1956 and 1971, at what is now Memorial Sloan-Kettering Cancer Center, Dr. Willet Whitmore experimented with various isotopes including ^{222}Radon, ^{192}Iridium, and ^{125}Iodine [7]. Dr. Whitmore ultimately described a well-tolerated technique in which ^{125}Iodine was sealed in titanium cylinders and implanted using a retropubic approach. However, the necessity for an open approach offered little advantage to the prostatectomy, and it was not until 1983 when Dr. Holm from Denmark described transrectal ultrasound (TRUS)-guided ^{125}I placement that the advantages to brachytherapy were realized [8].

Experience with brachytherapy has expanded rapidly since the introduction of TRUS and template guidance over 30 years ago, and now nearly a century after the first brachytherapy experiments, brachytherapy has become a simple, minimally invasive and well-tolerated option for the management of localized prostate cancer. Advantages to modern brachytherapy include rapid post-procedure

M.C. Ward, M.D. • J.P. Ciezki, M.D.
K.L. Stephans, M.D. (✉)
Department of Radiation Oncology,
Taussig Cancer Institute, Cleveland Clinic
Foundation, 9500 Euclid Avenue, Desk T28,
Cleveland, OH 44195, USA
e-mail: STEPHAK@ccf.org

recovery, relatively low morbidity, low cost, and excellent long-term control rates. Brachytherapy is a standard therapeutic option for patients with clinically localized disease and is recognized by various national and international organizations including NCCN, NCI, ACS, AUA, ASTRO, and EORTC among others. This chapter reviews the modern indications and techniques for the performance of brachytherapy.

Evaluation

The pre-procedure evaluation for a patient considered a candidate should be similar to those undergoing other definitive localized therapies such as surgery or external beam radiotherapy (EBRT). This includes a thorough history and physical focusing on previous genitourinary or pelvic surgeries (including transurethral resection of the prostate), previous radiotherapy, use of anticoagulants, medical conditions associated with increased risk with anesthesia, and radiation-related complications (i.e., active lupus, scleroderma, or inflammatory bowel disease). Special attention should be paid to urinary symptoms—practitioners may find the IPSS (International Prostate Symptom Score) to be a useful validated system to document pre-procedure function. Laboratory components of the workup should include a recent PSA (prostate-specific antigen) and pathologically confirmed prostatic carcinoma with Gleason scoring. For intermediate and particularly high-risk patients a metastatic workup including a bone scan and CT imaging of the abdomen and pelvis may be indicated. Preanesthesia evaluation typically includes complete blood count, complete metabolic profile, coagulation studies, and a urinalysis. Further advanced testing may be indicated to investigate any potential anesthesia risks identified during the standard evaluation.

Patient Selection

Patient selection is perhaps the most critical step to performing prostate brachytherapy. A number of organizations including the American Brachytherapy Society (ABS), American College of Radiology (ACR), and the American Society for Radiation Oncology (ASTRO) have published recommendations for the selection of brachytherapy candidates [9, 10], though institutional practices in experienced centers may allow for selection both within and beyond these fundamental guidelines.

Patient-related factors to consider include a patient's age, medical comorbidities and associated life expectancy, pelvic anatomy, surgical history, and pre-implant urinary symptoms. Age and comorbidities should be considered as in any therapy for prostate cancer whereby those at low risk of prostate cancer mortality during their expected lifetime should strongly consider active surveillance. Patients who are obese may be comparatively best suited for brachytherapy, as prostatectomy may be complicated and they are at increased operative and perioperative risk, while their body habitus may challenge external beam image guidance, dosimetry, and table limits.

Care should be taken in patients who may be at high risk for post-implant toxicity. These include a high IPSS score or a post-void residual of more than 100 cm^3 [9]. ABS guidelines define "high" IPSS score as greater than 20 although recent Radiation Therapy Oncology Group (RTOG) trials exclude scores persisting above 15 [11] despite the use of alpha-blockers. Such patients may benefit from prostatectomy as this may relieve obstructive or irritative symptoms, whereas radiation (and in particular brachytherapy) may elicit at least short-term exacerbation of these symptoms [1]. If such patients are adequately counseled regarding the risk of exacerbation, the potential for dependence upon intermittent straight catheterization, and a future TURP, the procedure may be performed.

Relative contraindications to brachytherapy such as a previous history of TURP and a large prostate are also manageable with experience. A prior history of TURP may make the procedure more technically challenging as it limits some positions that could be used for source placement. Additionally it may predict for urinary incontinence after brachytherapy based on the initial experience in Seattle, Washington [12], though this has been challenged in the recent literature [13]. TURP also poses technical challenges for other treatment options such as prostatectomy by potentially making the surgical anastomosis more challenging. Patients with history of TURP should be considered on a case-by-case basis as the size and anatomy of the TURP can vary significantly and counseled for potential risk of incontinence when proceeding with brachytherapy.

The ABS guidelines consider prostate size greater than 60 cm^3 to be a potential contraindication [14]. With the implantation of larger prostates one might encounter pubic arch interference during an implant; however, with patient positioning and needle technique this can typically be overcome in our experience. Flexion of the patient's hips (to open the pubic arch), flattening of the probe angle, and needle insertion at a medial and inferior grid coordinate with a lateral and upward needle angle all help overcome arch interference. Likewise, the number of sources required increases linearly with prostate volume although there is no known maximum threshold. In our experience, biochemical outcomes are significantly improved with larger glands, though some series do suggest slightly higher acute urinary retention rates [15, 16].

Hesitation may be necessary when a patient presents with a history of prior pelvic irradiation although after consideration, brachytherapy may be the ideal option provided the patient and disease factors support the risk of treatment, given that pelvic adhesions may inhibit the surgical approach and external beam radiation may expose significantly more tissue to reirradiation and the associated potential for toxicity.

Disease-related factors are generally grouped according to the NCCN risk stratification. Low-risk patients, those with a Gleason score of 6, PSA less than 10 ng/mL, and T1-T2a clinical stage, are ideal candidates for brachytherapy with biochemical outcomes at least equal to other available treatment modalities [17, 18].

Intermediate-risk patients, those with a Gleason score of 7, PSA 10–20 ng/mL, or T2b-T2c clinical stage, also appear to be good candidates for implant alone. ABS guidelines have recommended caution in approaching these patients with brachytherapy as monotherapy as intermediate-risk (and high-risk) patients may have a higher prevalence of extraprostatic extension (EPE), seminal vesicle invasion (SVI), or nodal spread, all of which may place the patient at risk of failure with brachytherapy implant alone. Despite this, an increasing volume of data supports the notion that brachytherapy alone can achieve equivalent outcomes to other modalities for intermediate-risk prostate cancer and in our center this is a routine treatment option (Fig. 8.1) [17, 19, 20]. The use of brachytherapy monotherapy in high-risk patients, those with a Gleason of ≥8, PSA above 20 ng/mL, or T3 disease, is investigational as these patients have historically not been considered candidates for brachytherapy alone. Select experiences have shown encouraging results with HDR or LDR brachytherapy [21, 22] though this is not a standard treatment option for high-risk disease. Many institutions combine EBRT with androgen deprivation, with or without brachytherapy boost in these patients [23]. This has been associated with favorable outcomes in some series; however it needs to be approached with caution due to increased risk of toxicity in this group [17, 19]. Of particular concern, RTOG 00-19 examined the role of EBRT to 45 Gy in 25 fractions followed 2–6 weeks later by an ^{125}I boost of 108 Gy in 183 intermediate-risk prostate cancer patients [24]. The 8-year estimated rate of grade 3 and higher GU and GI toxicity was 15 %, including two patients with grade 4 bladder necrosis. This reported toxicity is significantly higher than that seen in other similar select single-institution studies and emphasizes that caution should be taken in considering patients for combined EBRT and brachytherapy. The presence of confirmed lymph node metastasis or other metastatic disease is a contraindication to brachytherapy.

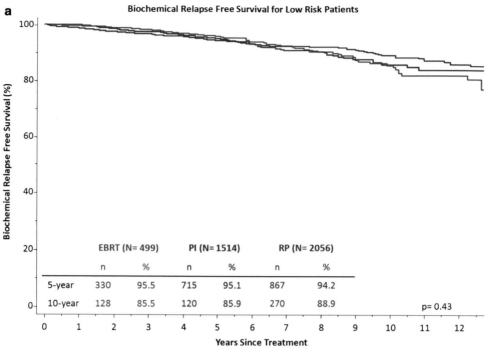

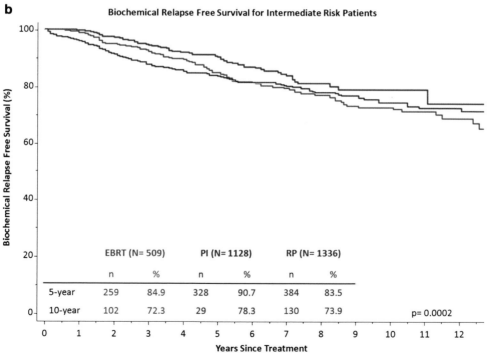

Fig. 8.1 Cleveland Clinic institutional outcomes by NCCN risk category between 1996–2014. Part (**a**) is low-risk, part (**b**) intermediate-risk and part (**c**) high risk. The number at-risk at 5 and 10 years along with the biochemical relapse free survival is listed in each table. Radical prostatectomy (RP) is shown in read, permanent implant (PI) listed in blue and external beam radiotherapy (EBRT) listed in green

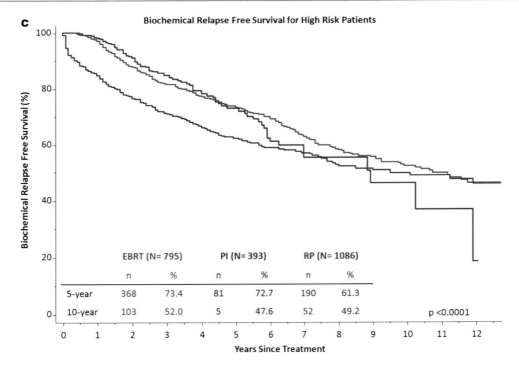

Fig. 8.1 (continued)

Personnel and Roles

To perform brachytherapy safely and efficiently a multidisciplinary team is necessary which may include the urologist, radiation oncologist, medical physicist, radiation therapist, anesthesiologist, and perhaps a medical dosimetrist. Furthermore, prostate brachytherapy has been shown to have a significant learning curve and therefore referral to a team experienced in prostate brachytherapy is recommended [25–27].

If brachytherapy is the recommended procedure, involvement of a medical physicist is necessary. Medical physicists are trained and certified in the planning, calibration, delivery, and quality control of radiotherapy. Their role is critical to the appropriate calculations required to deliver the radiation dose prescribed by the physician. A radiation therapist qualified in the handling and delivery of radiotherapy can aid in the logistical challenges inherent to radioactive sources as well as catheter loading during the procedure.

Anesthesia is recommended in the performance of brachytherapy although the type and delivery are institution specific. General anesthesia is most often used although some institutions prefer spinal anesthesia and obtain excellent outcomes. Local anesthesia with or without sedation is also possible although it requires an experienced physician and, while generally well tolerated, is occasionally more uncomfortable for the patient [28].

Radiation Biology and Physics

A basic understanding of radiation biology and physics can be useful when participating in the planning and the delivery of brachytherapy. Two broad categories of dose delivery can be identified: low dose rate (LDR) and high dose rate (HDR). LDR implants typically deliver dose at a rate of 0.01–2 Gy per hour and require weeks to months to reach full dose. HDR implants may deliver dose at a rate greater than 12 Gy per hour and require only minutes to deliver full dose to the target. LDR brachytherapy for prostate cancer is typically given via permanent seed implants using isotopes of [103]Palladium, [125]Iodine, or [131]Cesium elements. HDR implants in the modern era typically employ [192]Iridium via a remote

Table 8.1 Physical properties of various elements used in prostate brachytherapy

Element	Avg. photon energy (keV)	Method of decay	Half-life (days)	Initial Estimated dose rate (cGy/h)
[103]Palladium	21	EC	17	21.2
[125]Iodine	28	EC	59	7.0
[131]Cesium	29	EC	9.7	34.2
[192]Iridium	398	β^- (95 %) and EC	73.8	>1,200
[198]Gold	412	β^-	2.7	107

afterloader. HDR brachytherapy as monotherapy is considered investigational by many investigators [29]. Table 8.1 lists various elements used in prostate brachytherapy for comparison.

Measurement of Dose

Various methods for quantification of ionizing radiation dose are available and a general familiarity is necessary for the clinician comparing various techniques in radiotherapy, particularly between EBRT and prostate brachytherapy. The most clinically relevant measure of radiation dose today is the Gray (Gy) which is the SI unit of absorbed dose and defined as 1 Joule (J) of energy deposited per kilogram of tissue (J/kg). The rad, previously the standard, is equivalent to 0.01 Gy, or 1 cGy. Gray is a measure of energy deposited in tissue and has various biological effects dependent on a myriad of other factors. The sievert (Sv) is a unit defined as the human biologic equivalent or effective dose and is most relevant in radiation safety applications. For photons, 1 Gy is approximately equal to 1 Sv. Protons, having an increased mass and an increased relative biologic effectiveness, deliver approximately 2 Sv per 1 Gy absorbed. The rem (Röntgen equivalent in man), a previous standard, is equivalent to 1 rad or 1 cGy. It is important to remember that the biologic effective dose (BED) is a complex comparison particularly when made between brachytherapy and EBRT. The clinical BED is most related to the fraction size and number of fractions delivered but is also related to the quality of radiation (energy, photon vs particles such as protons), dose rate, the type of tissue in question, the rate of cellular repair, oxygenation, and the cell-cycle state of the tumor. The complexity

of these comparisons explains the challenges encountered when attempting to identify the ideal radiotherapeutic approach to prostate cancer.

Dose Deposition: Energy and the Inverse Square Law

The energy of ionizing radiation is a key factor in determining the depth of tissue penetration. Higher energy photons travel further into tissue before attenuating as defined by the percent depth–dose (PDD) curve. Early kilovoltage units used for EBRT were ineffective in treating prostate cancer due to the inability to deposit dose deep into the pelvis. The key advantage of brachytherapy over EBRT is quantified by the "inverse square law" which states that the intensity of radiation emitted from a source is inversely proportional to the square of the distance from the source (8.1). This allows for relatively high doses to the tissue in contact with the source and a much lower dose to the normal tissue surrounding the target.

Inverse Square Law

$$\text{Dose}(r) \propto \frac{1}{r^2}, \qquad (8.1)$$

where r = distance from source.

Treatment Planning and Dosimetry

Target Volume Delineation

Regardless of the technique used for delivering prostate brachytherapy, the target and the organs at risk (OARs) remain the same. The prostate, including the capsule and a margin surrounding the capsule, is the key target for localized disease.

For intermediate and high-risk disease the proximal 1–2 cm of the seminal vesicles may be included in the target volume. Key OARs include the urethra, bladder, rectum, and penile bulb. It is not possible to deliver sufficient dose to the pelvic lymph nodes with transperineal prostate brachytherapy.

Contouring

"Contouring," a common term in the field of radiation oncology, is the process by which targets and OARs are identified on imaging in order to calculate dose delivered to the structure. While automated algorithms exist, contours are always checked and edited by the physician. The urologist, radiation oncologist, and medical physicist vary in their degree of involvement in contouring based on institution and physician preference. The RTOG has assembled an expert panel to define an atlas of standardized references for contouring [30].

Generally the prostate should be contoured as the key target, sometimes coined the "gross tumor volume" (GTV) although it may be more appropriate to describe the prostate as the "clinical target volume" (CTV) as it is a volume concerning for disease which is not entirely composed of cancerous tissue. Some may describe a "planning target volume" (PTV) which, by strict definition, is an expansion on the CTV accounting for motion or set-up error. Given that brachytherapy is performed under real-time visualization of the target this standard definition of PTV is of debatable importance in the brachytherapy setting and is more applicable to EBRT. Many centers however do target an expansion of the prostate to account for risk of extracapsular extension which in surgical series appears to be within 4 mm in more than 90 % of cases [31, 32]. If an expansion is applied this may vary by NCCN risk group, but is typically approximately 5 mm at the apex and base, 2–3 mm anteriorly and laterally with no expansion on the posterior border. This could be considered part of the CTV, or otherwise PTV.

For ultrasound-based planning techniques commonly applied intraoperatively, images are sent from the ultrasound probe to the contouring

Table 8.2 Example of dosimetric goals for LDR and HDR brachytherapy

	Monotherapy prescription	Prescription with EBRT
^{125}I	144–160 Gy	110–125 Gy
^{103}Pd	108–110 Gy	90–100 Gy
^{192}Ir	6–7 Gy×6 fractions [33–36]	9–15 Gy×1 fraction [37, 38]
	12–13.5 Gy×2 fractions [39]	5.5 Gy×3 fractions [40, 41]

	Preplan	Post-plan
V100	100 %	90 % Ideal, acceptable 80 %
V150	<50 %	<50 %
V200	<20 %	<20 %
D90	115 % (110–130 %)	100 %
Urethra D_{max}	<150 % (ideally <120 %)	<150 %
Rectum D_{max}	<1 cm^3 receiving 100 %	<1 cm^3 receiving 100 %

software. The physician is then able to contour the edges of the prostate to define the CTV as well as the bladder or rectum as necessary. Any desired expansion can be easily performed at this time. After contouring, a plan can be generated which specifies a seed arrangement which best meets the targeted metrics (Table 8.2). For CT-based HDR plans or post-implant dosimetry verification scans the rectum is typically contoured from the rectosigmoid junction to the level of the anal verge. The peritoneal reflection and true rectosigmoid junction are difficult to delineate on imaging and therefore typically defined as the level where the colon begins to deviate laterally on axial imaging and begins to lose a circular shape. The bladder should be distended and the wall from the dome to the bladder neck should be included. The penile bulb, which is difficult to visualize on CT imaging without contrast, catheterization, or MRI fusion, begins inferiorly to the apex of the prostate and originates posterior to the urethra, having a circular shape in this region. Although debatable, some studies have related the dose delivered to the penile bulb to the risk of erectile dysfunction [42, 43]. The penile bulb contour should not extend to the pendulous portion of the penis. Small bowel and femoral heads are not typically of concern in brachytherapy and receive only background dose.

Dose Prescription

After selecting and contouring the CTV and PTV, dose is prescribed to cover the intended target volume. For LDR monotherapy, common dose prescriptions include 144–160 Gy for ^{125}I and 110–125 Gy for ^{103}Pd. For a combined modality approach, the dose is typically 108–110 Gy for ^{125}I, 90–100 Gy for ^{103}Pd, and 10–22.5 Gy in 1–3 fractions for HDR (although no consensus in HDR dosing has been reached) [44]. Typical planning goals for ^{125}I monotherapy include a preplanned D90 (minimum dose to 90 % of the PTV) between 110 and 130 % of the prescribed dose to reach a post-plan goal of 100 %. The preplanned V100 (volume receiving 100 % of the prescribed dose) should approach 100 % (at least >99 %) to obtain a post-plan V100 of at least 80 %, though ideally greater than 90 %. Regarding OARs, the maximum urethral dose should be less than 150 % of the prescribed dose (our institution target is less than 120 %) and the volume of the rectum receiving the prescription dose should be less than one cubic centimeter [45–47]. These dosimetric goals are summarized in Table 8.2. Figure 8.2 shows an example of a TRUS-guided preplan and the resulting post-implant evaluation on CT.

Isotope Selection

As stated in Table 8.1, there are various properties inherent to each isotope. Selection between LDR isotopes is based primarily on institution preference and there is debate in the literature regarding any potential clinical benefit of palladium, iodine, or cesium [48]. Iodine may have a logistical and cost-saving benefit as the half-life is extended and excess seeds can be saved for future procedures. The low dose rate of iodine allows for very low radiation exposure to personnel performing the procedure but may lead to a longer duration of sequelae. The decreased half-life of palladium potentially reduces the duration of sequelae and allows the option of implantation prior to EBRT in the setting of combined

therapy. A randomized trial comparing ^{125}I to ^{103}Pd found no difference in biochemical outcome or long-term toxicity while suggesting a greater peak but faster resolution of acute effects with ^{103}Pd as one might expect from the dose rate [49]. Theories of a low alpha/beta ratio for prostate cancer suggest that cesium may have a tumor control benefit due to increased rate of dose deposition although no clear clinical data support this [50]. Iridium is the element of choice for HDR brachytherapy.

Planning: Intraoperative vs. Preoperative

Planning of radiation dosimetry can be accomplished before, during, or after the implant procedure is performed. If the planning is accomplished days to weeks before the procedure, this is termed preplanning and has the logistical benefit of estimating the seed count although organ motion may be an issue. Intraoperative planning can be performed before the implant (intraoperative preplanning) or simultaneous with the implant (interactive intraoperative planning). With HDR brachytherapy treatment planning is performed postoperatively via CT performed with the implant in place and radiation is delivered via remote afterloader. Advantages to the preoperative technique include logistical flexibility and decreased time under anesthesia. The intraoperative preplanning technique, preferred by our institution, allows for accurate planning of the sources without significant interference of organ motion or deformation and improves dosimetric parameters compared to a preplanning technique [51]. If performed efficiently the increase in time under anesthesia is minimal. Post-planning with HDR brachytherapy has the potential advantage of optimization of source dwell times, allowing for some adjustment of the dose distribution after the implant. Despite this, implant (needle or catheter) position is critical and cannot be completely overcome by source optimization alone. If preoperative or intraoperative planning is performed, a postoperative verification scan is necessary.

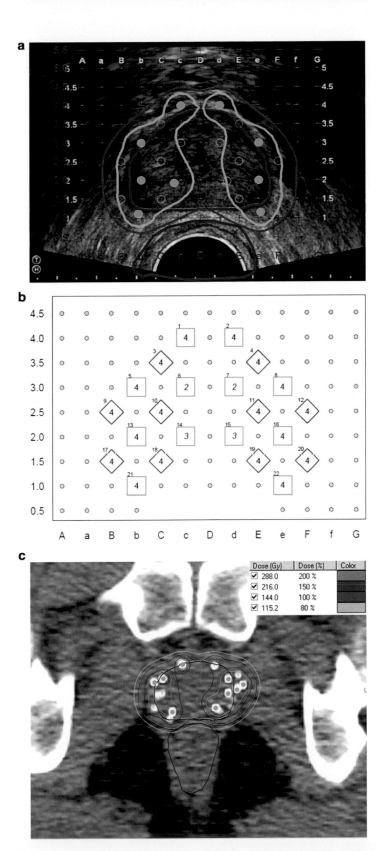

Fig. 8.2 TRUS-guided preplan and the resulting post-plan evaluation by CT. Isodose lines represent varying levels of radiation deposition. (**a**) TRUS-guided preplan showing the prostate CTV (*red*) with the 100 % isodose line (*purple*) and 150 % isodose line (*light blue*) with seed locations superimposed on the template grid (*green*). Note the urethral and rectal sparing. (**b**) TRUS-guided template showing needle spacing. (**c**) Axial post-plan by CT. (**d**) Coronal post-plan by CT. (**e**) Sagittal post-plan by CT. (**f**) 3D reconstruction depicting seeds within prostate in comparison to the contoured bladder and rectal volumes

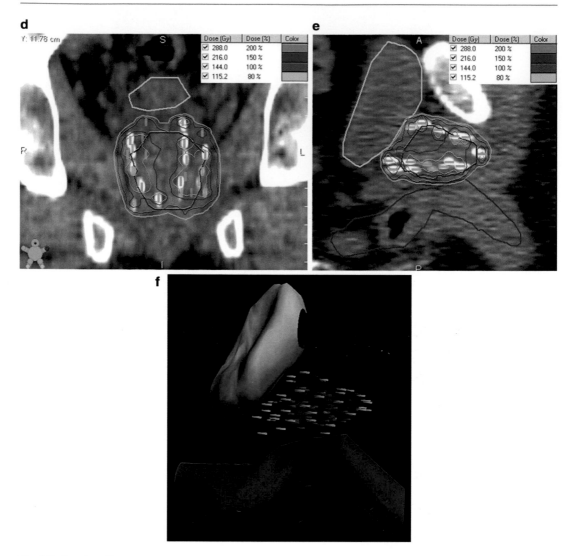

Fig. 8.2 (continued)

Dosimetry and Planning: LDR vs. HDR Brachytherapy

HDR brachytherapy varies slightly in dosimetry and technique from LDR brachytherapy. During LDR brachytherapy permanent seeds are implanted whereas during HDR brachytherapy temporary catheters are placed (via the same TRUS-guidance technique) before the radioactive source is administered via remote afterloader. This technique eliminates the potential for seed migration or embolization and eliminates dose to treating staff. Another advantage is the ability to confirm the quality of the implant after the catheters have been placed but prior to radiation delivery. HDR can potentially deliver a more homogeneous dose profile due to post-planning and a higher energy of ^{192}Ir is compared to the LDR isotopes (Table 8.2) [52]. A third potential radiobiologic advantage includes the hypofractionated schedule which may have a disease-control benefit based on the theories of a low alpha/beta ratio as mentioned above. Despite these advantages, careful technique is still required to ensure a high-quality implant. One potential disadvantage is the increased volume of normal tissue receiving low doses of radiation. The major disadvantage, however, is that most current schedules call for multiple implantation procedures (or for the implant to remain in place for an extended period of time over multiple fractions) as the use of single-fraction HDR monotherapy or boost remains investigational [53]. Ultimately, while there are multiple potential advantages to HDR brachytherapy, long-term randomized trials with patient-reported outcomes are yet to be conducted; therefore, brachytherapy technique remains the physician and institution's choice.

Implantation Technique

LDR Technique

Procedural techniques will vary according to institution and type of implant required. Here a typical LDR implant using an intraoperative preplanning technique is described.

Prior to the procedure patients are encouraged to undergo routine preparation including avoidance of aspirin and anticoagulants for 5 days and abstaining from eating the night before. A bowel preparation using a Fleet enema or comparable can be helpful and is routinely administered 1 h prior to the procedure in our practice. Perioperative antibiotics are routine and typically include a cephalosporin or fluoroquinolone as indicated.

In the operating room the patient is placed in the exaggerated dorsal lithotomy position. Routine clean-contaminated surgical preparation is indicated. A complete surgical drape is institution specific but in our opinion is unnecessary. Ultrasound jelly placed into the rectum following rectal irrigation can be helpful prior to ultrasound placement. The TRUS unit should be capable of providing axial as well as sagittal images and include a stabilization device with template guidance. A template is attached to the TRUS unit to allow for accurate catheter insertion. Urethral visualization is usually possible with ultrasound and it is unnecessary to use a Foley catheter in the majority of cases. The use of a Foley can obstruct the view of the anterior prostate. If the urethra is unable to be visualized, consider injection of a small amount of either lubricant jelly or air if clinically necessary.

The entire prostate from 1 cm proximal to the base to 1 cm distal to the apex is imaged with 5 mm axial slices and images are sent to the planning software. The length, width, and height of the prostate are measured and volume is calculated both by the ultrasound unit and by the planning software. Correlation with the length of the prostate on sagittal view and the number of axial slices should be ensured to avoid error (e.g., a 4 cm prostate length should yield approximately 8–9 slices of prostate, 12–13 total captured slices).

Following image acquisition, commercially available planning software is then used to contour the CTV and OARs as detailed above. After calculation of the seed distribution, a final plan will display the number of sources and needles necessary and the correlated insertion location on the grid attached to the TRUS unit. At this point, ensure that the preplanned isodose lines are appropriate and that the preplan dosimetric goals have been met. Linked seeds ensure accurate separation and have been shown to decrease the rate of migration and embolization [54, 55]. Linked seeds should be used in the periphery with loose seeds inserted centrally near the urethra to allow for spontaneous or cystoscopic removal of a single source should such a situation arise. Likewise, we routinely use loose seeds for the inferior medial perirectal seeds as a precaution. Brachytherapy plans should typically be symmetrical and follow a modified peripheral loading technique [56].

During implantation under axial guidance (Fig. 8.3a), insert the needle through the template and firmly into the perineum. Begin with the needle in the axial coordinate farthest from the TRUS probe as image distortion may increase if the seeds are first delivered near the probe. An increased speed of needle insertion will minimize deflection of the needle. The deflection of the needle is related to the direction of the bevel and can be used to adjust for error. Once the needle is within the target coordinate, switch to a sagittal view to guide the depth as necessary. This use of sagittal ultrasound imaging eliminates the need for fluoroscopy in guiding the depth of needle insertion. Next, visualize the bladder wall and insert the needle in to the prostate base (Fig. 8.3b). At this point you will feel the increased resistance of the prostate capsule and also visually see increased deflection of the prostate on ultrasound. Once depth of insertion has been confirmed,

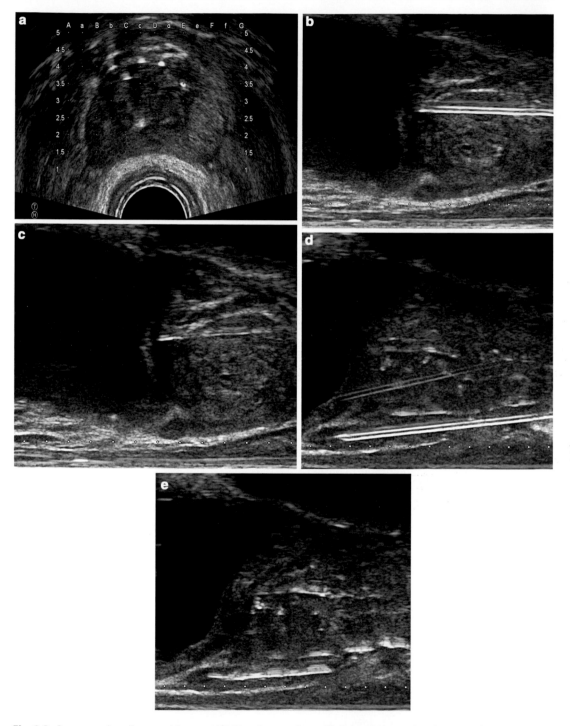

Fig. 8.3 Intraoperative ultrasound images. (**a**) Template grid superimposed on the prostate on axial TRUS with needle insertion at coordinate E, 3.5. (**b**) Needle inserted in to the base of the prostate abutting the bladder wall as visualized on sagittal ultrasound imaging. (**c**) After removal of the needle in (**b**) the strand of seeds remains in place. (**d**) Sagittal image showing a needle tangential to the rectal wall. This technique is acceptable provided the seeds are implanted deep enough not to be deployed into the wall itself. (**e**) After the stranded seeds are deployed they rest in the prostate and seminal vesicle volume with a clear margin on the rectal wall

deploy the seeds by holding the stylet in place and removing the needle (Fig. 8.3c). Ensure that the needle is not inserted further during the process of deploying the seeds as the bladder wall may be implanted. When inserting the inferior, perirectal needles extreme caution must be used to avoid deploying a source in, or immediately adjacent to the rectum. While it is occasionally necessary to pass a needle through the rectum for some patients, this can typically be avoided by inserting the needle into a higher than intended grid location and then guiding the needle inferiorly during insertion to avoid the rectal wall (Fig. 8.3d, e). A careful understanding of how this effects dosimetry is important and should be considered during planning. During placement we routinely use this technique for patients with steep rectal angles.

HDR Technique

The technique used for the implantation of HDR catheters is similar to the technique used when implanting permanent LDR sources. The catheters are inserted via the same TRUS-guided template technique described above although the catheters are left in place and the spacing may be wider due to the increased energy of ^{192}Ir. Following implantation of the catheters, the placement is confirmed via either TRUS, CT, or MRI. This scan is then used for planning purposes and the typical OARs are contoured. It is critical that the catheters remain in place once the planning has begun, as any displacement may result in dosimetric error. Once structures are contoured, inverse planning may be applied to optimize the dwell times of the ^{192}Ir source. Once the plan is complete, it is sent to the remote afterloader which is connected to the catheters. The treatment time varies by implant but is approximately 10 min.

Difficult Cases

Occasionally the delivery of the prescribed plan may be technically challenging. With proper technique and experience, almost no case need be aborted. Pubic arch interference, one of the most common challenges, can typically be avoided via an exaggerated lithotomy position as increasing hip flexion removes the pubic arch from the path of the needle and allows for direct access to the prostate from the perineum. If pubic arch interference remains an issue a more medial and inferior insertion position is selected and the needle's bevel adjusted to track superior and laterally. If needed a finger or other tool can be placed between the perineum and the template to further guide and deflect the needle. A slower insertion speed will increase the degree of deflection. Attempts at insertion should be kept to a minimum as the risk of prostatic hematoma increases as more attempts are made.

Post-procedure Management and Acute Toxicity

After completion of the implant cystoscopy may play a role in evaluating the urethra and bladder wall for improperly placed seeds. Some institutions choose to perform cystoscopy routinely while others choose only to pursue cystoscopy if blood is present at the urethral meatus and does not clear with irrigation. In coordination with the institution's radiation safety guidelines, a survey meter is used to screen any fluid leaving the patient. Measurements necessary may vary; however, exposure 1 m from the patient after implant must be less than one millirem per hour for discharge. Exposure is negligible to routine contacts who may come near a patient in the first weeks although it is recommended that small children do not spend extended time in the lap of a patient in the first 2–3 months following LDR implant (no more than 20 min out of a 3 h period repetitively). Implant activity is considered negligible after a period of five half-lives has passed (approximately 85 days for ^{103}Pd and 295 days for ^{125}I).

Acute toxicity from brachytherapy is typically modest. Acute toxicity is dominated by temporary urinary irritative and obstructive symptoms as well as fatigue, though may also include prostatitis, dysuria, urinary obstruction, or proctitis. Upon discharge it is recommended to provide an antibiotic regimen for 7–10 days. An α-blocker such as tamsulosin is recommended for 2–6 months or until urinary symptoms resolve to ameliorate urinary obstruction due to radiation-induced edema. Rarely catheterization may be necessary for patients experiencing urinary obstruction. We strongly recommend self-catheterization with a straight catheter rather than an indwelling Foley in order to minimize discomfort and risk of infection. Pain is usually minimal with a mild analgesic rarely necessary. Four weeks after LDR implant the patient should return for a CT scan to evaluate the quality of the implant. Commercially available software is used to identify the seeds and estimates the dose distribution. The prostate and OARs are delineated as above. If areas with insufficient dose are identified one should consider their clinical significance, and if needed they may be reimplanted with supplemental seeds at this time.

Quality of Life, Late Toxicity, and Management

The severity and frequency of late toxicity from brachytherapy is a frequent topic of debate in the literature. The variance in the incidence of erectile dysfunction, dysuria, cystitis, and radiation proctitis among physician-reported cohorts highlights the role for patient-reported outcomes in future studies. The largest study of patient-reported outcomes comparing quality of life between EBRT, prostatectomy, and brachytherapy is the 2008 ProstQA study reported in the *New England Journal of Medicine* [1]. In this study prostatectomy was associated with a relative detriment in sexual function and incontinence scores. EBRT and brachytherapy were associated with better preservation of continence and sexual function while causing more significant acute urinary obstruction (which ultimately returned towards baseline), as well as mild bowel irritation. Factors which independently predicted changes in quality of life and satisfaction for brachytherapy patients included increased age, increased initial PSA, hormonal therapy, EBRT boost, Gleason score less than 7, and prostate size.

The management of late complications from brachytherapy including dysuria, urinary obstruc-

tion, urethral stricture, cystitis, or proctitis typically requires a multidisciplinary approach. Dysuria may relate to prostatitis, cystitis, or urethritis. Infectious etiologies should be excluded. For supportive care mild symptoms of dysuria, urgency, or frequency, medical management is possible with medications such as tamsulosin, pyridium, oxybutynin, tolterodine, pentosan, hyoscyamine, or belladonna/opium suppositories. A transient flare in obstructive symptoms is common but the majority return to baseline IPSS score and greater than 90 % of patients return to baseline within 1 year [57]. Urethral stricture or chronic obstruction is uncommon and can be managed endoscopically. Chronic radiation cystitis presenting as hematuria is rare after brachytherapy and may require bladder irrigation and cystoscopy with coagulation. Radiation proctitis presents as rectal urgency or bleeding and on colonoscopy appears as erythema or friability localized to the anterior rectal wall. Medical management may include sucralfate, steroid enemas, or 5-ASA compounds such as sulfasalazine. Endoscopic management of rectal bleeding with 4 % formalin or argon plasma coagulation appears equivalent [58]. Randomized evidence also exists for the benefit of hyperbaric oxygen to accelerate the healing process inhibited by radiation-induced injury to the microvasculature [59]. Biopsy of the irradiated rectum should be judicious to avoid possible fistula formation. If necessary to exclude second malignancy or inflammatory bowel disease, biopsy should be directed towards the lateral or posterior rectal wall. The incidence of Grade 3 late toxicity after brachytherapy is variable in the literature but in the modern era is expected to be on the order of 5–10 % for any genitourinary toxicity and 1–5 % for any gastrointestinal toxicity [57, 60–63]. Less than one percent of patients will require formalin for rectal bleeding and 0.3 % will develop a fistula [62]. With experienced users extremely low rates of toxicity are reported with 10 year grade 2 or higher GU and GI toxicity in only 4.3 and 1.7 % percent of patients treated at the Cleveland Clinic, respectively (Fig. 8.4) [60].

The development of a radiation-induced second malignancy of the pelvis is a theoretical

a

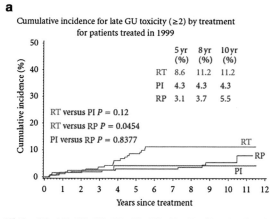

Cumulative incidence for late GU toxicity (≥2) by treatment
for patients treated in 1999

	5 yr (%)	8 yr (%)	10 yr (%)
RT	8.6	11.2	11.2
PI	4.3	4.3	4.3
RP	3.1	3.7	5.5

RT versus PI P = 0.12
RT versus RP P = 0.0454
PI versus RP P = 0.8377

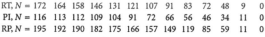

	0	1	2	3	4	5	6	7	8	9	10	11	12
RT, N =	172	164	158	146	131	121	107	91	83	72	48	9	0
PI, N =	116	113	112	109	104	91	72	66	56	46	34	11	0
RP, N =	195	192	190	182	175	166	157	149	119	85	59	11	0

b

Cumulative incidence for late GI toxicity (≥2) by treatment
for patients treated in 1999

	5 yr (%)	8 yr (%)	10 yr (%)
RT	7.8	7.8	7.8
PI	1.7	1.7	1.7
RP	0	0	0

RT versus PI P = 0.0081
RT versus RP P = 0.0002
PI versus RP P = 0.154

	0	1	2	3	4	5	6	7	8	9	10	11	12
RT, N =	172	161	153	144	131	123	113	95	87	76	56	13	0
PI, N =	116	115	114	110	106	92	73	67	57	46	34	10	0
RP, N =	195	195	194	186	180	170	161	151	122	88	61	11	0

Fig. 8.4 Long-term Grade 2 or higher toxicity comparisons between radical prostatectomy, permanent seed implant, and external beam radiotherapy at the Cleveland Clinic Foundation in 1999 [59]. Reprinted from Hunter GK, Reddy CA, Klein EA, et al. Long-term (10-year) gastrointestinal and genitourinary toxicity after treatment with external beam radiotherapy, radical prostatectomy, or brachytherapy for prostate cancer. Prostate Cancer. 2012;2012:853487

concern of radiotherapy although incidence is likely very small. SEER data for all patients receiving radiotherapy estimated the risk of radiation-induced second malignancy to be roughly 0.5 % [64]. One series found age and smoking to be independent predictors of second malignancy after prostate radiotherapy while the use of radiotherapy over surgery was not [65].

Posttreatment Surveillance, Biochemical Recurrence, and the PSA Bounce

Recent NCCN guidelines for routine prostate cancer surveillance include a PSA every 6–12 months for 5 years then annually with a digital rectal examination every year which may be omitted if the PSA is undetectable [66]. A PSA measured every 6 months appears optimal in the detection and surveillance of brachytherapy patients [67]. The upper age limit when surveillance becomes unnecessary is not specified and left to clinical judgment.

Biochemical recurrence after radiotherapy has been a topic of debate in the past decades. The original RTOG consensus defined recurrence as three consecutive rises in PSA above the post-treatment nadir [68]. However, this definition is very dependent upon the number and timing of PSAs taken, and the 2006 RTOG "Phoenix" definition of a rise in PSA by more than 2 ng/mL is more widely accepted today [69]. Androgen recovery should be considered in patients after discontinuing antiandrogen therapy.

The "PSA bounce," defined as an increase in PSA greater than 0.2 ng/mL than the nadir followed by a decrease to or below the initial nadir, is a known phenomenon following prostate brachytherapy and occurs in roughly 46 % of patients [70]. This can occur despite androgen deprivation therapy and is more common in younger patients. PSA bounce most commonly occurs within the first 3 years of implant (median 15 months), and close PSA follow-up should be considered for patients with a PSA rise within this timeframe without other clinical evidence of recurrent disease.

Conclusion

Brachytherapy is a straightforward outpatient procedure and is an option for patients with clinically localized prostate cancer offering cure rates comparable to other treatment options. Treatment results primarily in acute GU irritation and obstruction, with a very low long-term toxicity profile. There is debate in the literature regarding the optimal techniques in patient selection and treatment delivery although experience is critical to minimize complications. Ultimately, patient selection is driven by clinical risk and the toxicity profile of each modality, whereas brachytherapy technique is driven by physician preference and institutional experience. Future directions in prostate brachytherapy include optimization of treatment planning, measurement of patient reported outcomes, and healthcare value analyses.

References

1. Sanda MG, Dunn RL, Michalski J, et al. Quality of life and satisfaction with outcome among prostate-cancer survivors. N Engl J Med. 2008;358(12): 1250–61.
2. Dam H. The New Marvel in Photography. McClure's Mag. 1896;6:403.
3. Curie M, Curie M, Bemont G. Sur une nouvelle substance fortement radioactive contenue dans la pechblende. Compt Rend Acad Sci (Paris). 1898;127: 1215–7.
4. Pasteau O. Traitement du cancer de la prostate par le radium, par le Dr Octave Pasteau. Impr. de H. Gaignault: Issoudun; 1911.
5. Young HH. The use of radium in cancer of the prostate and bladder. J Am Med Assoc. 1917; LXVIII(16):1174–7.
6. Flocks RH, Kerr HD, Elkins HB, Culp D. Treatment of carcinoma of the prostate by interstitial radiation with radio-active gold (Au 198): a preliminary report. J Urol. 1952;68(2):510–22.
7. Whitmore Jr WF, Hilaris B, Grabstald H. Retropubic implantation to iodine 125 in the treatment of prostatic cancer. J Urol. 1972;108(6):918–20.
8. Holm HH, Juul N, Pedersen JF, Hansen H, Stroyer I. Transperineal 125iodine seed implantation in prostatic cancer guided by transrectal ultrasonography. J Urol. 1983;130(2):283–6.
9. Nag S, Bice W, DeWyngaert K, Prestidge B, Stock R, Yu Y. The American Brachytherapy Society recommendations for permanent prostate brachytherapy postimplant dosimetric analysis. Int J Radiat Oncol Biol Phys. 2000;46(1):221–30.
10. Rosenthal SA, Bittner NH, Beyer DC, et al. American Society for Radiation Oncology (ASTRO) and American College of Radiology (ACR) practice guideline for the transperineal permanent brachytherapy of prostate cancer. Int J Radiat Oncol Biol Phys. 2011;79(2):335–41.
11. RTOG 0815. A phase III prospective randomized trial of dose-escalated radiotherapy with or without short-term androgen deprivation therapy for patients with intermediate-risk prostate cancer. 2012. http://www.rtog.org/ClinicalTrials/ProtocolTable/StudyDetails.aspx?study=0815. Accessed 16 Nov 2013.
12. Blasko JC, Ragde H, Grimm PD. Transperineal ultrasound-guided implantation of the prostate: morbidity and complications. Scand J Urol Nephrol Suppl. 1991;137:113–8.
13. Salembier C, Rijnders A, Henry A, Niehoff P, Andre Siebert F, Hoskin P. Prospective multi-center dosimetry study of low-dose Iodine-125 prostate brachytherapy performed after transurethral resection. J Contemp Brachytherapy. 2013;5(2):63–9.
14. Davis BJ, Horwitz EM, Lee WR, et al. American Brachytherapy Society consensus guidelines for transrectal ultrasound-guided permanent prostate brachytherapy. Brachytherapy. 2012;11(1):6–19.
15. Quan AL, Ciezki JP, Reddy CA, et al. Improved biochemical relapse-free survival for patients with large/wide glands treated with prostate seed implantation for localized adenocarcinoma of prostate. Urology. 2006;68(6):1237–41.
16. Stone NN, Stock RG. Prostate brachytherapy in men with gland volume of 100cc or greater: technique, cancer control, and morbidity. Brachytherapy. 2013; 12(3):217–21.
17. Grimm P, Billiet I, Bostwick D, et al. Comparative analysis of prostate-specific antigen free survival outcomes for patients with low, intermediate and high risk prostate cancer treatment by radical therapy. Results from the Prostate Cancer Results Study Group. BJU Int. 2012;109 Suppl 1:22–9.
18. Zelefsky MJ, Yamada Y, Pei X, et al. Comparison of tumor control and toxicity outcomes of high-dose intensity-modulated radiotherapy and brachytherapy for patients with favorable risk prostate cancer. Urology. 2011;77(4):986–90.
19. Sylvester JE, Grimm PD, Wong J, Galbreath RW, Merrick G, Blasko JC. Fifteen-year biochemical relapse-free survival, cause-specific survival, and overall survival following I(125) prostate brachytherapy in clinically localized prostate cancer: Seattle experience. Int J Radiat Oncol Biol Phys. 2011; 81(2):376–81.
20. Vassil AD, Murphy ES, Reddy CA, et al. Five year biochemical recurrence free survival for intermediate risk prostate cancer after radical prostatectomy, external beam radiation therapy or permanent seed implantation. Urology. 2010;76(5):1251–7.

21. Taussig Cancer Institute. 2012 Outcomes. 2012. http://my.clevelandclinic.org/Documents/outcomes/2012/outcomes-cancer.pdf. Accessed 8 Dec 2012.

22. Yoshioka Y, Konishi K, Sumida I, et al. Monotherapeutic high-dose-rate brachytherapy for prostate cancer: five-year results of an extreme hypofractionation regimen with 54 Gy in nine fractions. Int J Radiat Oncol Biol Phys. 2011;80(2):469–75.

23. D'Amico AV, Moran BJ, Braccioforte MH, et al. Risk of death from prostate cancer after brachytherapy alone or with radiation, androgen suppression therapy, or both in men with high-risk disease. J Clin Oncol. 2009;27(24):3923–8.

24. Lawton CA, Yan Y, Lee WR, et al. Long-term results of an RTOG Phase II trial (00-19) of external-beam radiation therapy combined with permanent source brachytherapy for intermediate-risk clinically localized adenocarcinoma of the prostate. Int J Radiat Oncol Biol Phys. 2012;82(5):e795–801.

25. Lee WR, deGuzman AF, Bare RL, Marshall MG, McCullough DL. Postimplant analysis of transperineal interstitial permanent prostate brachytherapy: evidence for a learning curve in the first year at a single institution. Int J Radiat Oncol Biol Phys. 2000; 46(1):83–8.

26. Taussky D, Moumdjian C, Larouche R, et al. Seed migration in prostate brachytherapy depends on experience and technique. Brachytherapy. 2012;11(6): 452–6.

27. Bockholt NA, Deroo EM, Nepple KG, et al. First 100 cases at a low volume prostate brachytherapy institution: learning curve and the importance of continuous quality improvement. Can J Urol. 2013;20(5): 6907–12.

28. Wallner K. Prostate brachytherapy under local anesthesia; lessons from the first 600 patients. Brachytherapy. 2002;1(3):145–8.

29. Zaorsky NG, Doyle LA, Hurwitz MD, Dicker AP, Den RB. Do theoretical potential and advanced technology justify the use of high-dose rate brachytherapy as monotherapy for prostate cancer? Expert Rev Anticancer Ther. 2014;14(1):39–50.

30. Gay HA, Barthold HJ, O'Meara E, et al. Pelvic normal tissue contouring guidelines for radiation therapy: a Radiation Therapy Oncology Group consensus panel atlas. Int J Radiat Oncol Biol Phys. 2012;83(3): e353–62.

31. Davis BJ, Pisansky TM, Wilson TM, et al. The radial distance of extraprostatic extension of prostate carcinoma: implications for prostate brachytherapy. Cancer. 1999;85(12):2630–7.

32. Sohayda C, Kupelian PA, Levin HS, Klein EA. Extent of extracapsular extension in localized prostate cancer. Urology. 2000;55(3):382–6.

33. Demanes DJ, Martinez AA, Ghilezan M, et al. High-dose-rate monotherapy: safe and effective brachytherapy for patients with localized prostate cancer. Int J Radiat Oncol Biol Phys. 2011;81(5):1286–92.

34. Jabbari S, Weinberg VK, Shinohara K, et al. Equivalent biochemical control and improved prostate-specific antigen nadir after permanent prostate seed implant brachytherapy versus high-dose three-dimensional conformal radiotherapy and high-dose conformal proton beam radiotherapy boost. Int J Radiat Oncol Biol Phys. 2010;76(1):36–42.

35. Lee B, Shinohara K, Weinberg V, et al. Feasibility of high-dose-rate brachytherapy salvage for local prostate cancer recurrence after radiotherapy: the University of California—San Francisco experience. Int J Radiat Oncol Biol Phys. 2007;67(4):1106–12.

36. Rogers CL, Alder SC, Rogers RL, et al. High dose brachytherapy as monotherapy for intermediate risk prostate cancer. J Urol. 2012;187(1):109–16.

37. Morton GC, Loblaw DA, Sankreacha R, et al. Single-fraction high-dose-rate brachytherapy and hypofractionated external beam radiotherapy for men with intermediate-risk prostate cancer: analysis of short- and medium-term toxicity and quality of life. Int J Radiat Oncol Biol Phys. 2010;77(3):811–7.

38. Pistis F, Guedea F, Pera J, et al. External beam radiotherapy plus high-dose-rate brachytherapy for treatment of locally advanced prostate cancer: the initial experience of the Catalan Institute of Oncology. Brachytherapy. 2010;9(1):15–22.

39. Ghilezan M, Martinez A, Gustason G, et al. High-dose-rate brachytherapy as monotherapy delivered in two fractions within one day for favorable/intermediate-risk prostate cancer: preliminary toxicity data. Int J Radiat Oncol Biol Phys. 2012;83(3):927–32.

40. Martinez AA, Demanes DJ, Galalae R, et al. Lack of benefit from a short course of androgen deprivation for unfavorable prostate cancer patients treated with an accelerated hypofractionated regime. Int J Radiat Oncol Biol Phys. 2005;62(5):1322–31.

41. Chen YC, Chuang CK, Hsieh ML, et al. High-dose-rate brachytherapy plus external beam radiotherapy for T1 to T3 prostate cancer: an experience in Taiwan. Urology. 2007;70(1):101–5.

42. Mendenhall WM, Henderson RH, Indelicato DJ, Keole SR, Mendenhall NP. Erectile dysfunction after radiotherapy for prostate cancer. Am J Clin Oncol. 2009;32(4):443–7.

43. Roach 3rd M, Nam J, Gagliardi G, El Naqa I, Deasy JO, Marks LB. Radiation dose-volume effects and the penile bulb. Int J Radiat Oncol Biol Phys. 2010;76(3 Suppl):S130–4.

44. Kotecha R, Yamada Y, Pei X, et al. Clinical outcomes of high-dose-rate brachytherapy and external beam radiotherapy in the management of clinically localized prostate cancer. Brachytherapy. 2013;12(1):44–9.

45. Waterman FM, Dicker AP. Probability of late rectal morbidity in 125I prostate brachytherapy. Int J Radiat Oncol Biol Phys. 2003;55(2):342–53.

46. Mueller A, Wallner K, Merrick G, et al. Perirectal seeds as a risk factor for prostate brachytherapy-related rectal bleeding. Int J Radiat Oncol Biol Phys. 2004;59(4):1047–52.

47. Tran A, Wallner K, Merrick G, et al. Rectal fistulas after prostate brachytherapy. Int J Radiat Oncol Biol Phys. 2005;63(1):150–4.

48. Kollmeier MA, Pei X, Algur E, et al. A comparison of the impact of isotope (((125)I vs. (103)Pd) on toxicity and biochemical outcome after interstitial brachytherapy and external beam radiation therapy for clinically localized prostate cancer. Brachytherapy. 2012;11(4): 271–6.

49. Herstein A, Wallner K, Merrick G, et al. I-125 versus Pd-103 for low-risk prostate cancer: long-term morbidity outcomes from a prospective randomized multicenter controlled trial. Cancer J. 2005;11(5):385–9.

50. Brenner DJ, Hall EJ. Fractionation and protraction for radiotherapy of prostate carcinoma. Int J Radiat Oncol Biol Phys. 1999;43(5):1095–101.

51. Wilkinson DA, Lee EJ, Ciezki JP, et al. Dosimetric comparison of pre-planned and or-planned prostate seed brachytherapy. Int J Radiat Oncol Biol Phys. 2000;48(4):1241–4.

52. Wang Y, Sankreacha R, Al-Hebshi A, Loblaw A, Morton G. Comparative study of dosimetry between high-dose-rate and permanent prostate implant brachytherapies in patients with prostate adenocarcinoma. Brachytherapy. 2006;5(4):251–5.

53. Hoskin P, Rojas A, Ostler P, et al. High-dose-rate brachytherapy alone given as two or one fraction to patients for locally advanced prostate cancer: acute toxicity. Radiother Oncol. 2014;110(2):268–71.

54. Eshleman JS, Davis BJ, Pisansky TM, et al. Radioactive seed migration to the chest after transperineal interstitial prostate brachytherapy: extraprostatic seed placement correlates with migration. Int J Radiat Oncol Biol Phys. 2004;59(2):419–25.

55. Al-Qaisieh B, Carey B, Ash D, Bottomley D. The use of linked seeds eliminates lung embolization following permanent seed implantation for prostate cancer. Int J Radiat Oncol Biol Phys. 2004;59(2):397–9.

56. Sylvester JE, Grimm PD, Eulau SM, Takamiya RK, Naidoo D. Permanent prostate brachytherapy preplanned technique: the modern Seattle method step-by-step and dosimetric outcomes. Brachytherapy. 2009;8(2):197–206.

57. Keyes M, Miller S, Moravan V, et al. Urinary symptom flare in 712 125I prostate brachytherapy patients: long-term follow-up. Int J Radiat Oncol Biol Phys. 2009;75(3):649–55.

58. Yeoh E, Tam W, Schoeman M, et al. Argon plasma coagulation therapy versus topical formalin for intractable rectal bleeding and anorectal dysfunction after radiation therapy for prostate carcinoma. Int J Radiat Oncol Biol Phys. 2013;87(5):954–9.

59. Clarke RE, Tenorio LM, Hussey JR, et al. Hyperbaric oxygen treatment of chronic refractory radiation proctitis: a randomized and controlled double-blind crossover trial with long-term follow-up. Int J Radiat Oncol Biol Phys. 2008;72(1):134–43.

60. Hunter GK, Reddy CA, Klein EA, et al. Long-term (10-year) gastrointestinal and genitourinary toxicity after treatment with external beam radiotherapy, radical prostatectomy, or brachytherapy for prostate cancer. Prostate Cancer. 2012;2012:853487.

61. Tanaka N, Asakawa I, Anai S, et al. Periodical assessment of genitourinary and gastrointestinal toxicity in patients who underwent prostate low-dose-rate brachytherapy. Radiat Oncol. 2013;8:25.

62. Price JG, Stone NN, Stock RG. Predictive factors and management of rectal bleeding side effects following prostate cancer brachytherapy. Int J Radiat Oncol Biol Phys. 2013;86(5):842–7.

63. Zelefsky MJ, Yamada Y, Cohen GN, et al. Intraoperative real-time planned conformal prostate brachytherapy: post-implantation dosimetric outcome and clinical implications. Radiother Oncol. 2007; 84(2):185–9.

64. Berrington de Gonzalez A, Curtis RE, Kry SF, et al. Proportion of second cancers attributable to radiotherapy treatment in adults: a cohort study in the US SEER cancer registries. Lancet Oncol. 2011;12(4): 353–60.

65. Zelefsky MJ, Pei X, Teslova T, et al. Secondary cancers after intensity-modulated radiotherapy, brachytherapy and radical prostatectomy for the treatment of prostate cancer: incidence and cause-specific survival outcomes according to the initial treatment intervention. BJU Int. 2012;110(11):1696–701.

66. NCCN Clinical Practice Guidelines. Prostate Cancer Version 4.2013, 7/26/2013. 2013. www.nccn.org. Accessed 16 Nov 2013.

67. Caloglu M, Ciezki JP, Reddy CA, et al. PSA bounce and biochemical failure after brachytherapy for prostate cancer: a study of 820 patients with a minimum of 3 years of follow-up. Int J Radiat Oncol Biol Phys. 2011;80(3):735–41.

68. Consensus statement: guidelines for PSA following radiation therapy. American society for therapeutic radiology and oncology consensus panel. Int J Radiat Oncol Biol Phys. 1997;37(5):1035–41.

69. Roach 3rd M, Hanks G, Thames Jr H, et al. Defining biochemical failure following radiotherapy with or without hormonal therapy in men with clinically localized prostate cancer: recommendations of the RTOG-ASTRO Phoenix Consensus Conference. Int J Radiat Oncol Biol Phys. 2006;65(4):965–74.

70. Ciezki JP, Reddy CA, Garcia J, et al. PSA kinetics after prostate brachytherapy: PSA bounce phenomenon and its implications for PSA doubling time. Int J Radiat Oncol Biol Phys. 2006;64(2):512–7.

Prostate Cryoablation

9

Timothy Byler and Imad Nsouli

Introduction

In 2008, 214,633 men in the United States were diagnosed with cancer of the prostate. Despite this high incidence, 28,471 men died from prostate cancer which accounts for about 7 % of the group [1]. This contrast raises debate on the need for treatment and how to select those patients who should be treated. In the recently published PIVOT trial, patients were randomized between observation and prostatectomy for localized prostate cancer. In 10-year follow-up, surgery did not significantly reduce mortality when compared to observation [2]. For those patients who desire treatment against advise for observation or have features that suggest treatment should be offered, minimally invasive modalities are attractive while lowering the possibility of side effects. In this respect, prostate cryotherapy and high intensity-focused ultrasound are being further investigated.

T. Byler, M.D.
Department of Urology, SUNY Upstate Medical University, 750 East Adams Street, Syracuse, NY 13210, USA

I. Nsouli, M.D. (✉)
Department of Urology, SUNY Upstate Medical University, 750 East Adams Street, Syracuse, NY 13210, USA

Urology Division, Surgery Department, VA Medical Center, Syracuse, NY, USA
e-mail: nsoulii@upstate.edu

The concept of using cold therapy to remedy disease has been described as far back as Ancient Egypt. In the 1840s, James Arnott used salt solutions containing crushed ice to freeze advanced cervical and breast cancers [3]. Through these early uses, Arnott noted that tissue that had been chilled developed a white, hard appearance and hemorrhaging ceased [4]. As an appreciation for the chemical properties of various elements advanced at the turn of the twentieth century, contemporary cryoablation began to take form. The ability to solidify carbon dioxide gas occurred around 1900 along with its use in the treatment of dermatologic disease [5, 6]. A series of advancements in both medicine and chemistry lead to increasing understanding and applications of cold therapy. Excellent reviews of the development of cryotechnology can be found by Gage [7] and Rubinsky [4].

The first generation of modern prostate cryoablation emerged in the 1960s. Automated cryoablation probes were initially developed in 1961 by Cooper and Lee. These were designed for brain tumors, and used a liquid nitrogen-based cooling system [4]. This was adapted by Gonder in 1964 for use in prostatic disease. Originally by using the canine prostate and later using transurethral freezing in humans, they were able to show the response of tissue to freezing [8]. This was done through a urethral freezing probe and monitored with digital rectal examination. The interest generated by these original reports led to further work using an open transperineal approach by Flock [9] and a closed transperineal approach by Megallil [10].

R.V. Khanna et al. (eds.), *Surgical Techniques for Prostate Cancer*,
DOI 10.1007/978-1-4939-1616-0_9, © Springer Science+Business Media New York 2015

These procedures were prior to intraoperative imaging modalities and control of the propagating ice ball was difficult. This led to unacceptable complications including urethral sloughing and urethrorectal fistula formation, limiting the application of cryoablation.

Largely discarded until the 1980s, interest in prostate cryosurgery was renewed with several innovations [11]. The introduction of real-time monitoring with transrectal ultrasound allowed clinicians to control the ice ball generated and lower involvement of surrounding structures. The next modification was the transition from a liquid nitrogen-based system to a gas system which allowed smaller probe diameters. This relied on the Joule-Thompson principal which will be discussed later. Finally, urethral preservation using a urethral warming catheter further lowered rates of urethral sloughing and incontinence post-procedure. An excellent review of these advancements with details can be found by Saliken and associates [11].

Cryobiology

The methods of cellular death when cold therapy is applied have been heavily studied in efforts to control cancer death while minimizing surrounding tissue destruction. With his original work in 1964, Gonder [8] showed the pathology of his treatments. The mechanisms of cellular death in the canines undergoing cryoablation included:

1. Cellular dehydration and toxic electrolyte concentrations
2. Crystallization and rupture of cellular membranes
3. Protein denaturing
4. Vascular stasis
5. Thermal Shock

Over the next 40 years, these principals have largely remained unchanged with emphasis on certain elements.

Tissue Response to Freezing

The glands of the prostate are surrounded by a stroma rich in smooth muscle and vasculature [12]. This interaction plays a central role in the effects of cells to thermal injury. The accumulation of solute, elevation of cellular pH, destabilization of cellular membranes, and mechanical sheering by ice formation lead to cell death when cryoablation is performed. Around tissue temperatures of 0 °C, the extracellular fluid begins to crystalize [11]. This crystallization leads to an accumulation of solute within the remaining extracellular fluid and induces osmotic shifts based on differential concentrations. The results of this shift lead to accumulation of electrolytes and toxins normally dilute in the cell to more dangerous levels. This accumulation leads to damage to the enzymatic machinery and destabilization of the cellular membranes. As enzymatic systems are unable to operate, pH changes lead to protein breakdown. Around −15 °C, intracellular ice begins to form. The formation of ice both extracellular and intracellular leads to a mechanical sheering of cellular membranes and direct disruption [13].

The vascular injury from freezing is also important to outcome. Research into cellular death following frostbite has provided a higher understanding of the vascular components in cryoablative death. Direct microvascular death, particularly venous, leads to tissue hypoxia and lack of nutrient supply [14]. There is a vascular stasis and thrombosis following freezing of the vasculature that further extrapolates this process.

The end result of freezing is direct cellular death and subsequent apoptosis of remaining cells. This apoptotic mechanism has been linked to mitochondrial mechanisms with rises of levels of BAX without BCL-2 up-regulation. Other mechanisms of cellular apoptosis are likely to be involved and are being investigated [15].

Joule-Thompson Effect

The method of delivery of freezing temperatures has evolved in the recent past to allow the procedure to be controlled better and safer for the patient. This effect was initially described in 1852 describing the free expansion of gases in a vacuum. In modern cryotherapy, it describes the transfer of energy between gases and the prostate that allow for temperature changes.

As a gas changes its pressure, its own specific thermodynamics determine if it will warm or cool. At 20 °C (room temperature), all gases except hydrogen, helium, and neon cool on their expansion [16]. Modern systems use Argon as their freezing gas and helium as the warming gas. The gases used during cryoablation are under high pressure (3,000 psi) and as they circulate through the cryogenic probes, they are exposed to atmospheric pressure (15 psi) [11]. Due to the Joule-Thompson Effect, as argon enters the probes, it expands under the lower pressure causing the gas to cool. This cooling is transmitted to the probe and into the tissue causing freezing. The removal of thermal energy from the prostate into the expanding argon gas is the basis for this temperature drop. In the converse, helium warms with this process and therefore transfers heat to the tissue, warming the prostate.

Modifiable Procedural Dynamics

In the AUA best practice statement from 2008, Babaian described the modifiable factors to increase success of thermal ablation [15] (Table 9.1).

Procedure

Patient Selection

Cryoablation is a treatment option that is suitable for patients with localized prostate cancer and negative metastatic evaluation. It can be offered to men who are unable or unwilling to undergo other forms of therapy. It can be safely used in men with prior pelvic radiation or significant bowel disease (i.e., Crohn's disease) in which radical surgery is often complicated.

Table 9.1 Modifiable factors in thermal ablation

Factor	Comments
Freeze rate	Rapid freeze > Slow Freeze
	Cancer cells adapt to slow freeze
Temperature monitor	Strongly advises for monitor
Nadir temperature	Traditionally –40 °C was used
	Recommend –20 °C
Thaw rate	Recommend passive thaw
Freeze cycles	Double freeze-thaw cycle advocated

Men with negative metastatic evaluations, but high-risk features (PSA > 20, Gleason 8 or above) should be counseled about their risk of occult disease and offered lymph node dissection (AUA best practice) [15].

One of its major side effects is impotence and therefore it has been traditionally offered to men without potency or who are willing to lose potency.

Contraindications

Large prostate glands (>50 cm^3 traditional)
Prior transurethral resection of prostate, specifically within 3–6 months
Cancers within the transition or central prostate zones

Procedure

Preparation includes a liquid diet the day prior to the procedure and a bowel preparation to cleanse the rectum. An enema is given the morning of the procedure.

Patients are given a first generation cephalosporin prior to the procedure. The procedure is performed under general or spinal anesthesia. They are placed in dorsal lithotomy position. The perineum and penis should be prepped completely with all hair removed from the perineum.

Most cryotherapy rectal probes are mobile and attach to the underside of the operative table. Once the patient is positioned, the rectal probe is inserted and the prostate is visualized. A brachytherapy grid is placed against the perineum. It is our practice to place two anchor needles once the grid is placed (Fig. 9.1).

Probe placement sites are marked on the ultrasound screen. We ensure a distance of less than one centimeter between the probe sites and the prostate capsule, and a distance of less than 2 cm between probes. Seven probes are usually used. For small glands, five probes can be used. Two probes are placed at the apex of the prostate, two in the mid portion, and 3 at the base. The probes are placed under ultrasound guidance in both axial and sagittal views (Fig. 9.2). Sagittal view is used to ensure the bladder is not penetrated.

Fig. 9.1 Initial insertion of the transrectal ultrasound and grid

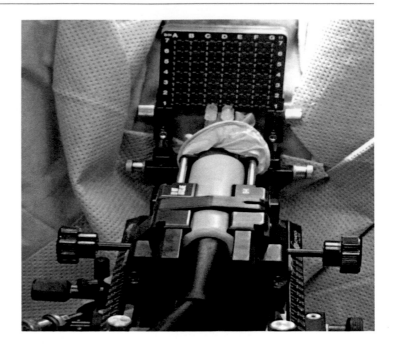

Fig. 9.2 (**a**) Transrectal ultrasound showing probe position. (**b**) Sagittal view showing expected probe locations. *Note*: *Numbers* correlate to freeze order, not probe number. *White lines* represent urethral catheter but probes are similar. *U* marks the urethra

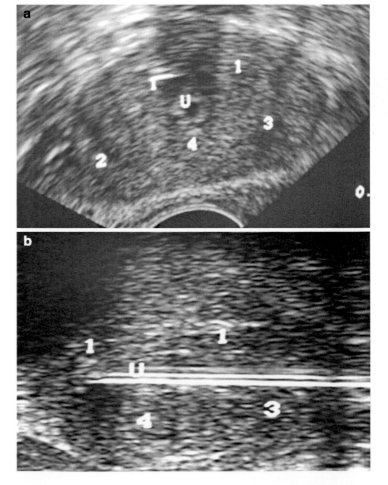

Once all probes are in place, the temperature probes are then placed. We use five temperature probes that will allow monitoring of the freeze process and of vital structures. One probe is placed at each neurovascular bundle, one at the apex, one at the external urinary sphincter, and one at Denonvillier's fascia.

A flexible cystoscopy is then performed to ensure there has been no violation of the urethra or bladder neck by any of the probes. It is our preference to use a suprapubic catheter as it is more comfortable to patients and allows monitoring of post-void residuals. It is inserted at this point. A guide wire is inserted via the scope into the bladder. The guide wire is left in place while the scope is removed and is used to help the insertion of the urethral warming catheter. The bladder is kept partially inflated during the procedure.

Two freeze-thaw cycles are completed in line with current recommendations. The temperature is brought down to −40 and held for 2 min. The temperature probes are monitored, and the ice ball is monitored using ultrasound guidance in both the sagittal and axial view. The freeze cycle is adjusted accordingly. Once an adequate ice ball is formed which involves the whole prostate, the freeze cycle is stopped and all probes are thawed. The process is then repeated for the second cycle. Once complete, the probes are removed and the urethral warming catheter is left while in the recovery area. It is removed about an hour later, and the patient is admitted overnight (Fig. 9.3).

Most patients have perineal bruising. They are discharged with scrotal support and suprapubic drainage for 7–10 days. A fluoroquinolone is given for the duration of the catheter placement.

Outcomes

Defining Cyrotherapy Success

A persistent problem with whole gland cryoablation has been the difficulty in defining adequate treatment. Whereas radical prostatectomy and radiation have guidelines for failure, such as rising PSA nadir, the ASTRO criteria, or the phoenix criteria, this does not exist for cryotherapy. In the 2010 updated AUA Best Practice Statement [15], the conclusion was "As a consequence, meaningful comparisons of these reported outcomes from radical prostatectomy and radiation therapy to cryosurgery are not possible." With this in mind, review of literature pertaining to whole gland ablation should be viewed with caution and should not be directly compared to other methods.

Filtering the available literature for mainly third generation cryogenic systems reveals a mixture of failure definitions. Most commonly used are the ASTRO and Phoenix criteria that were originally described for radiation (Table 9.2). Levy [17] examined the level of PSA nadir and its prediction of biochemical failure. Using the Cryo On-Line Registry (COLD), 2,427 patients were examined using PSA nadir cut-offs of less than 0.1 ng/mL, 0.1–0.5 ng/mL, 0.6–1.0 ng/mL, and 1.1–2.5 ng/mL. Increasing PSA nadir did show higher risk of treatment failure and the overall nadir was prognostic. Regardless of risk group, PSA nadir above 0.6 ng/mL was associated with significant 24-month biochemical failure. The authors caution that this cannot be used as a definition because the data was not correlated with disease-specific or metastatic-free survival.

In this regard, one study deserves special mention as it is one of the only direct comparison done prospectively, non-inferiority, and randomized. Published in Cancer 2010, Donnelley [18] performed a randomized trial comparing external beam radiation and primary whole gland cryoablation. All study patients did receive neoadjuvant hormone ablation with LH-RH agonist. They excluded patients who had bulky T3 tumor, previous radiation, previous hormone treatment, or had undergone TURP within the past 3 months. Primary endpoint was 36-month failure post-randomization using the phoenix definition. At primary end point, there was a 17 % failure in the cryoablation arm and 13 % in the external beam radiation arm. There had been 10 deaths from prostate cancer, 5 in each arm during the study with a disease-specific survival of 96 % for both treatment groups. The conclusion was that cryoablation was not inferior to external beam radiation for the treatment of localized prostate cancer.

Fig. 9.3 (a) Probes
inserted into perineum.
Appearance after all
probe are in place.
(b) Appearance of the
software. Temperature
and freeze times are
monitored with software

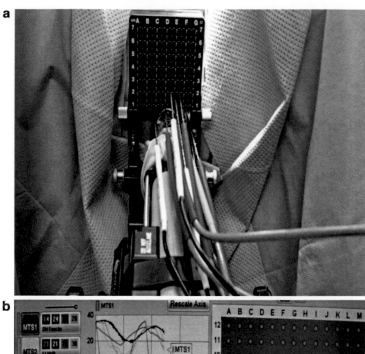

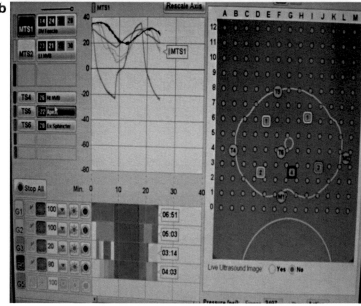

Table 9.2 Definitions of commonly used
criteria for biochemical failure

Criteria	Parameters
ASTRO	Three consecutive rises in PSA
Phoenix	PSA nadir + 2 ng/mL

erectile dysfunction, urethrorectal fistula formation, and incontinence. As the treatment modality
progressed, many of the features of our newest
cryoablation systems have been added specifically to prevent or limit these complications.

Primary Whole Gland Cryoablation

The gold standard in cryoablation is freezing
of the entire prostate gland. In the early work,
this method had significant morbidity including

Biochemical-Free Survival

Many studies have been published retrospectively reviewing cryoablation series with all
three cryogenic generation systems (Table 9.3).

Table 9.3 Publications of primary whole gland cryoablation using third generation systems

Publication	Patients	Follow-up	Definition	Overall BDFS (%)
Prepelica 2004	65	35 month	ASTRO	83
Hubosky 2007	89	1 year	ASTRO	94
Polascik 2007	50	18 month	PSA<0.5	90
Jones 2008	1,198	5 year	ASTRO	77

A brief review will be placed here with emphasis on the third generation argon-based systems. For a full review of many of the articles published, please refer to Levy [19].

The 10-year data available has been generated from mixed systems with both nitrogen and argon in use as the freezing agent. Cohen [20] used nitrogen-based system and retrospectively analyzed 204 patients finding a 10-year biochemical disease-free survival (BDFS) of 56 % using the ASTRO criteria and 62 % using the Phoenix criteria. When they further divided in risk groups, the Phoenix definition was 80, 74, and 45 % for low, moderate and high, respectively. Statistically, these groups were different by long-rank test.

Shorter term follow-up has been published by several groups. Polascik [21] analyzed 50 men undergoing third generation ablation with an 18-month follow-up. They reported a 90 % BDFS using a threshold PSA of 0.5. With a median follow-up of 35 months, Prepelica [22] used an argon-based system with 83 % BDFS using ASTRO criteria. Finally, with 89 patients undergoing third generation cryoablation, Hubosky [23] showed 94 % at 1-year follow-up. To address the small amount of data available, the COLD registry was developed. In 2008, Jones [24] published a series of 1,198 patients with 5-year data from the registry. These patients when stratified by risk group and using the ASTRO criteria showed 84, 73, and 75 % BDFS.

Overall, the short-term success of primary cryoablation ranges between 60 and 90 %. There are few studies examining the long term outcomes and less with consistent newer generation systems and failure definitions.

Complications of Whole Gland Cryoablation

Appropriate patient counseling of upcoming whole gland prostate cryoablation must include discussion of impotence, incontinence, urethrorectal fistula, chronic perineal pain, and urinary retention. Impotence occurs largely due to the proximity of the neurovascular bundles to the cryogenic probes and modern systems attempt to prevent this by neurovascular bundle temperature monitoring. Traditionally, series have shown large range of impotence rates, anywhere from 4 to 88 %, with most in the 50–80 % [25]. Due to the possibility of sphincter involvement, most series show a 0.4–15 % rate of incontinence. The possibility of neurologic injury with resultant chronic pelvic pain is reported 0.4–12 %. The dreaded complication of urethrocutaneous fistula is reported 1–2 % and is prevented by accurate temperature monitoring at denonvilliers fascia level. An excellent summary of key complications was published by Mourviev and Polascik [25].

Primary Focal Cryoablation

Focal cryoablation has become the subject of investigation within the past 10 years. As discussed earlier, traditionally a major side effect of whole gland cryoablation has been erectile loss. The concept of focal ablation would allow for preservation of the contralateral neurovascular bundles and therefore enhanced postoperative erectile function. Ideally this erectile preservation would not come at the expense of oncologic efficiency.

Table 9.4 Publications involving focal cryoablation

Publication	Pt	Follow-up	Template	Continence	Potency	Oncologic
Bahn [32]	31	70	Hemiablation	100	89	93
Onik [33]	55	43	Focal	98	85	94
Ellis [34]	60	15	Hemiablation	96	70	80
Lambert [35]	25	28	Hemiablation	100	71	88
Truesdale [36]	77	24	Hemiablation	100	100	73
Ward [30]	1,160	24	Variable	98	58	75

Multi-focality in Prostate Cancer

Focal ablation, cryoablation or high intensity-,focused ultrasound, represents the only current treatments for prostate cancer which do not treat the whole prostate gland. Prostate cancer multifocality therefore becomes an issue of paramount importance.

Initially in 1992, Villers [26] retrospectively reviewed prostatectomy specimens for mutlifocality. In the 234 radical prostatectomy specimens available in their review, 117 had only the index tumor present. The remaining 117 harbored 266 incidental tumors, which were under 0.5 mm in size on average. Thus, in their study, focal ablation would have missed many incidental tumors that may become recurrences. Using radical prostatectomy specimens, Mouraviev [27] showed that prostate cancer was unifocal in 20 % of cases, meaning that 1 in 5 men would be eligible for hemiablation while the remaining men had bilateral tumor. The significance of these incidental tumors has been studied by several groups as well. Noguuchi [28] evaluated 222 men with T1c-detected prostate cancer and classified them into three clinical groups—Unifocal, Multifocal tumor <0.5 mm, and multifocal >0.5 mm. Using this criteria, 76 % of their cohort had multifocal disease. After a follow-up of 52 months, 18 % of the cohort had biochemical recurrence mainly within the unifocal group. The authors concluded that the index tumor impacted overall biochemical survival. These findings have been collaborated by others [27, 29].

Templates in Focal Cryoablation

When considering a focal ablation, the choice of template and surrounding tissue destruction becomes important. Many templates have been proposed but, as can be seen in Table 9.4, only the hemi ablation template has published results as of yet. Ward [30] reviewed prostate specimens for applicability of two templates: hockey stick and hemiablation. In their review of 180 specimens with a unilateral positive biopsy preoperatively, they found that hemiablation would have treated 64 % of relevant cancer while hockey stick would have treated 81 %. They concluded that most dominant tumors would have been ablated and therefore focal ablation was a realistic possibility (Fig. 9.4).

Patient Selection

Focal cryoablation outcome depends on the quality of patient selection and that prostate cancer is indeed localized. The primary tumor must be treatable without damage to the neurovascular bundle or urinary sphincter. In a consensus article, Eggener [31] proposed rigid criteria for focal cryoablation consideration highlighting localized, low-grade disease with low percentage total cancer. Most published reports of focal cryoablation have been consistent with these guidelines, although the inclusion criteria are not as strict as those proposed by Eggener. As more data is available, these guidelines may broaden but for

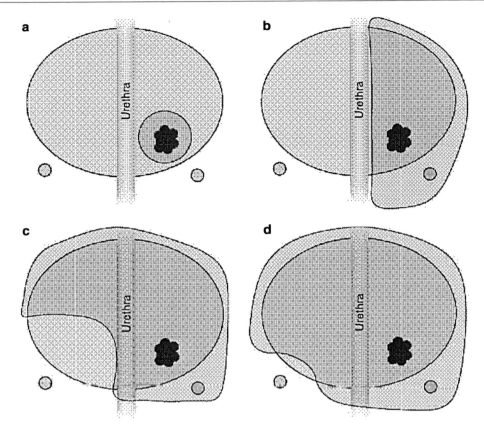

Fig. 9.4 Ablation templates for focal ablation. (**a**) Focal ablation, (**b**) hemiablation, (**c**) hockey stick ablation, (**d**) Sparing just the contralateral neurovascular bundle. From [37]. Reprinted with permission from Springer

now the only appropriate patients are those with low-risk disease and index tumor which is visible and localized.

Outcome Data

To date, there have been no published phase II or above clinical trials on focal cryoablation. The chart below (Table 9.4) shows the major works that are available with several outcome measures.

Majority of the trials agree that oncologic follow-up from 15 to 70 months is between 80 and 90 % biochemical-free survival. This is consistent with whole gland cryoablation. Considering the patient selection often used for these trials, it is likely that this is artificially raised and if the patient population were broadened, it may decrease. Each of these studies also utilizes different biopsy regimens and diagnostic tools. As expected, the potency and continence rates are enhanced from whole gland.

Conclusions

Cryoablation of the prostate has been around for many years and underwent many changes. In its current state, there continues to be a lack of long-term data to support long-term oncologic control. As series continue to mature, many of these questions will hopefully be answered. The ability to monitor and establish a definition of failure is lacking. The side effect profile continues to be dominated by impotence, although rates are improving. Focal therapy is a reasonable option to avoid the erectile problems but once again, data is very limited.

Acknowledgment Special thanks to Dr. Alosh Madala and Dr. Gillian Stearns for intraoperative photography.

References

1. U.S. Cancer Statistics Working Group. United States Cancer Statistics: 1999–2008 Incidence and Mortality Web-based report. Atlanta: Department of Health and Human Services, Centers for Disease Control and Prevention, and the National Cancer Institute; 2012.
2. Wilt TJ, et al. Radical Prostatectomy versus Observation for Localized Prostate Cancer. N Engl J Med. 2012;367(3):203–13.
3. Arnott J. Practical illustrations of the remedial efficacy of a very low or anaesthetic tempature. Lancet. 1850;2:257–9.
4. Rubinsky B. Cryosurgery. Annu Rev Biomed Eng. 2000;2:157–87.
5. Pusey WA. The use of carbon dioxide snow in the treatment of nevi and other lesions of the skin. J Am Med Assoc. 1907;49:371–7.
6. Bracco D. The historic development of cryosurgery. Clin Dermatol. 1990;8(1):1–3.
7. Gage AA. History of cryosurgery. Semin Surg Oncol. 1998;14:99–109.
8. Gonder MJ, Soanes WA, Smith V. Experimental prostate cryosurgery. Invest Urol. 1964;1(6):609–10.
9. Flocks RH, Nelson CMK, Boatman DL. Perineal cryosurgery for prostatic carcinoma. J Urol. 1972; 108:933–5.
10. Megalli MR, Gursel EO, Veenema RJ. Closed perineal cryosurgery in prostatic cancer. Urology. 1974; IV(2):220–2.
11. Salken JC, Donnelly BJ, Rewcastle JC. The evolution and state of modern technology for prostate cryosurgery. Urology. 2002;60(Suppl 2A):26–33.
12. Gartner LP, Hiatt JL. Color atlas of histology. 3rd ed. Baltimore: Lippincott Williams and Wilkins; 2000.
13. Hoffman NE, Bischof JC. The cryobiology of cryosurgical injury. Urology. 2002;60:40–9.
14. Baust JG, Gage AA, Robilottto AT, Baust JM. The pathophysiology of thermoablation: optimizing cryoablation. Curr Opin Urol. 2009;19:127–32.
15. Babaian RJ, Donnelly B, Bahn D, et al. Best practice statement on cryosurgery for the treatment of localized prostate cancer. J Urol. 2008;180:1993–2004.
16. Kyle BG. Chemical and process thermodynamics. 3rd ed. Upper Saddle River, NJ: Prentice Hall PTR; 1999.
17. Levy DA, Pisters LL, Jones JS. Primary cryoablation nadir prostate specific antigen and biochemical failure. J Urol. 2009;182:931–7.
18. Donnelly BJ, Saliken JC, Brasher PMA, Ernest SD, Rewcastle JC, Lau H, Robinson J, Trpkov K. A randomized trial of external beam radiotherapy vesus cryoablation in patients with localized prostate cancer. Cancer. 2010;116(2):323–30.
19. Levy D, Avallone A, Jones JS. Current state of urological cryosurgery: prostate and kidney. BJUI. 2010; 105:590–600.
20. Cohen JK, Miller RJ, Ahmed S, Lotz MJ, Baust J. Ten-year biochemical disease control for patients with prostate cancer treated with cryosurgery as primary therapy. Urology. 2008;71(3):515–9.
21. Polascik TJ, Nosnik I, Mayes JM, Mouraviev V. Short-term cancer control after primary cryosurgical ablation for clinically localized prostate cancer using third generation cryotechnology. J Urol. 2007;70(1): 117–21.
22. Prepelica KL, Okeke Z, Murphy A, Katz AE. Cryosurgical ablation of the prostate: high-risk patient outcomes. Cancer. 2005;103(8):1625–30.
23. Hubosky SG, Fabrizio MD, Schellhammer PF, Barone BB, Tepera CM, Given RW. Single center experience with third-generation cryosurgery for management of organ-confined prostate cancer: critical and evaluation of short-term outcomes, complications, and patient quality of life. J Endourol. 2007;21(12): 1521–31.
24. Jones JS, Rewcastle JC, Donnelly BJ, Lugnani FM, Pisters LL, Katz A. Whole gland primary cryoablation: initial results from the cryo on-line registry. J Urol. 2008;180:554–8.
25. Mouraviev V, Polascik TJ. Update on cryotherapy for prostate cancer in 2006. Curr Opin Urol. 2006;16: 152–6.
26. Villers A, Mcneal JE, Freiha FS, Stamey T. Multiple cancers in the prostate. Cancer. 1992;70(9):2313–8.
27. Mouraviev V, Villers A, Bostwick DG, Wheeler TM, Montironi R, Polascik TJ. Understanding the pathological features of focality, grade and tumour volume of early-stage prostate cancer as a foundation for parenchyma-sparing prostate cancer therapies: active surveillance and focal targeted therapy. BJU Int. 2011;108:1074–85.
28. Noguchi M, Stamey T, Mcneal JE, Nolley R. Prognostic factors for multifocal prostate cancer in radical prostatetectomy specimens: lack of significance of secondary cancers. J Urol. 2003;170: 459–63.
29. Wise AM, Stamey TA, McNeal JE, Clayton JL. Morphologic and clinical significance of multifocal prostate cancers in radical prostatectomy specimens. Urology. 2002;60:264–9.
30. Ward JF, Jones JS. Focal cryotherapy for localized prostate cancer: a report from the national Cryo On-Line Database(COLD) Registry. BJU Int. 2012; 109(11):1648–54.
31. Eggener SE, Scardino PT, Carroll PR, et al. Focal therapy for localized prostate cancer: a critical appraisal of rationale and modalities. J Urol. 2007;178:2260–7.
32. Bahn DK, Silverman P, Lee F, Badalament R, Bahn ED, Rewcastle JC. Focal prostate cryoablation: initial results show cancer control and potency preservation. J Endourol. 2006;20(9):688–92.
33. Onik G, Vaughan D, Lotenfoe R, Dineen M, Brady J. "Male Lumpectomy": focal therapy for prostate cancer using cryoablation. Urology. 2007;70:16–21.
34. Ellis DS, Manny TB, Rewcastle JC. Focal cryosurgery followed by penile rehabilitation as primary

treatment for localized prostate cancer: initial results. Urology. 2007;70:9–15.

35. Lambert EH, Bolte K, Masson P, Katz AE. Focal cryosurgery: encouraging health outcomes for unifocal prostate cancer. Urology. 2007;69(6): 1117–20.

36. Truesdale MD, Cheetham PJ, Hruby GW, Wenske S, Conforto AK, Cooper AB, Katz AE. An evaluation of patient selection criteria on predicting progression-free survival after primary focal unilateral nerve-sparing cryoablation for prostate cancer: recommendations for follow up. Cancer J. 2010;16(5):544–9.

37. Abern MR, Tsivian M, Polascik TJ. Focal therapy of prostate cancer: evidence-based analysis for modern selection criteria. Curr Urol Rep. 2012;13(2): 160–9.

Focal Ablation for Prostate Cancer   **10**

Julio M. Pow-Sang, Einar F. Sverrisson,
and Oscar M. Valderrama

Introduction

Prostate cancer is the second leading cause of cancer death in men in the United States. Since the introduction of PSA, there has been a progressive downward stage migration, with more new cases presenting as clinically localized, low volume, low grade disease. Ninety percent of all prostate cancers are found when the disease is confined to the prostate [1, 2].

Radical prostatectomy (RP) and radiation therapy (RT) aim to treat the whole prostate and seminal vesicles. Major side effects include urinary incontinence and erectile dysfunction in 5–20 % and 30–70 %, respectively [3]. While these sequelae have decreased with improvements in technique and technology, these morbidities have a significant impact on quality of life. PSA has contributed to the reduced prostate cancer mortality observed in the past decade, but at the same time increased the detection of potentially clinical insignificant cancers leading to overdiagnosis and overtreatment of some men [4]. The estimated overtreatment rate for prostate

J.M. Pow-Sang, M.D. (✉) • E.F. Sverrisson, M.D.
O.M. Valderrama, M.D.
Department of Genitourinary, Division of Oncology,
H. Lee Moffitt Cancer Center and Research Institute,
12902 Magnolia Drive, Tampa, FL 33612, USA
e-mail: Julio.powsang@moffitt.org

cancer is at least 30 % [5]. Men, who may have been overtreated for their early, potentially clinical insignificant disease, are at risk of lifelong morbidities derived from treatment.

In recent years focal therapy (FT) has emerged as a new alternative treatment for early prostate cancer. FT consists of completely ablating clinically significant cancer foci within the prostate while preserving normal tissue, the urinary sphincter, and the neurovascular bundles with the goal of minimizing side effects [4].

The selection of appropriate candidates for FT presents a challenge for the clinician. Prostate mapping biopsies and newer imaging technologies have been utilized to help select individuals with localized disease who may benefit from focal treatment.

Cryotherapy, high-intensity focus ultrasound (HIFU), Laser ablation, and photodynamic therapy (PDT) are current ablative modalities under investigation.

Diagnosis and Patient Selection for Focal Therapy

While the concept of focal therapy is simple, its application poses several challenges including optimal patient selection; localization, visualization, and characterization of significant cancer foci; accurate guidance of ablative energy in the area to be treated; follow-up and surveillance of untreated areas. A concern with FT is the multi-focality of prostate cancer as two thirds of patients with newly diagnosed prostate cancer present with more than one focus of cancer within the prostate. However, approximately 33 % will have unifocal tumor [6]. Additionally, approximately 40–80 % of multifocal tumors measure less than 0.5 mL in volume, which some investigators consider as clinically insignificant cancers [7–9]. This led to the concept of only treating the significant cancer foci (index lesion). Some reports conclude that the index lesion represents the main tumor volume, the highest Gleason score, and the potential site of extracapsular disease [2, 9].

At present, there is no agreement on which criteria should be applied for selecting optimal candidates for FT. Two multidisciplinary expert panels have reported on their selection criteria. Eggener et al. published the consensus of the International Task Force on Prostate Cancer and the Focal Lesion Paradigm (ITF-FLP) in 2007. They used clinical findings, biopsy, and imaging studies to define the criteria for patient selection. Clinical criteria included stage T1 or T2a, PSA less than 10 ng/mL, PSA density less than 0.15 ng/mL/cm^3, and PSA velocity less than 2 ng/mL yearly in the years prior to diagnosis. Biopsy criteria required obtaining a minimum of 12 cores and findings of a Gleason score 3 + 3 or less, less than 20 % of cancer in each core, and less than 33 % of total cores with cancer. Imaging criteria included single lesion with a maximum of 12 mm size, <10 mm of capsular contact, and no evidence of extraprostatic extension or seminal vesicle invasion [10]. In 2010, de la Rosette et al. published the consensus from an international expert meeting, the 2nd International Workshop on Focal Therapy, and Imaging in Prostate and Kidney Cancer (IWFTI). They concluded that patients appropriate for FT should have unilateral low to intermediate risk disease, clinical stage T2a or less, PSA <20 ng/mL, Gleason score 4 + 3 or less, and life expectancy of ten or more years. They recommended evaluation with transperineal mapping biopsies and excluded patients with anterior or apical tumors [11]. Other authors have reported that FT is suitable only for patients with low-risk disease (clinical stage T1c-T2a,

Gleason grade 3 + 3, and PSA < 10 ng/mL). Lindner et al. estimated that 45–85 % of patients fall into this category [12].

MRI technology is emerging as the most important imaging tool for identifying low-volume prostate cancers, assisting in risk stratification, and allowing for targeted biopsies [13, 14]. The sensitivity and specificity for identification of a significant cancer focus (>0.5 cm^3) was 86 % and 94 %, respectively [15]. MRI imaging remains the most important available imaging tool for identifying early prostate cancers and enabling focused use of energy ablative modalities.

Transperineal mapping biopsy (TPMB) has been proposed as a more accurate way to determine tumor focality and is being advocated as the preferred approach to select appropriate men for FT. Onik et al. compared the traditional biopsy technique to TPMB and found a large discrepancy [6, 16]. Barqawi et al. prospectively studied 3D mapping biopsy. They reported that a significant portion of men initially diagnosed with apparently low-risk disease harbored clinically significant cancer. These results demonstrate how 3D mapping biopsy may be applied to improve patient selection for FT [17].

Follow-Up After FT

After FT, verification of complete ablation of known cancer foci and detection of any de novo cancer in the untreated prostate gland should be assessed. Defining recurrence is another challenge evaluating the efficacy of focal therapy. As FT preserves prostatic tissue, PSA is not expected to become undetectable. Accepted criteria for biochemical recurrence after radiation therapy such as the ASTRO (three consecutive PSA rises after a nadir PSA) and Phoenix (nadir PSA + 2) criteria are not applicable to FT since they were not designed for use in this setting [5]. Despite no defined PSA cut point to evaluate treatment success, it is recommended that PSA should be continuously monitored during follow-up and rising PSA should be further investigated. Some investigators suggest defining biochemical failure as a PSA nadir + 50 % rise on follow-up [18].

Most investigators include post-treatment biopsy and imaging studies as part of their follow-up of patients treated with FT.

Focal Cryotherapy

Overview

Cryotherapy was initially reported in the 1960s by Cooper and Lee. They developed the first cryotherapy probe system using liquid nitrogen. The inclusion of urethral warmers, use of transrectal ultrasound (TRUS) for real time visualization of the ice ball, replacement of liquid nitrogen by argon gas for cooling and helium for warming, as well as thinner cryoneedles, allow surgeons for more accurate targeting enhancing its effectiveness while reducing potential side effects.

Initially cryotherapy was used to destroy the whole gland. More recently it has been investigated as a tool for FT. Focal cryotherapy is a modification of the standard technique, aiming to only treat the portion of the gland which has the clinically significant disease.

Mechanism of Action

The use of freezing temperatures and thawing cycles results in cell destruction by direct injury to the cells as well as secondary injury from the inflammatory response. The current technology uses argon gas flowing through hollow needles to freeze the prostate and helium gas to actively warm after freezing via the Joule-Thompson effect. There are three treatment parameters that correlate with cancer cell destruction: cooling rate, low temperature achieved, and duration of the freeze cycle.

After reaching a tissue temperature of less than 0 °C, the extracellular fluid starts to crystallize. Formation of crystals causes hyperosmotic pressure of the unfrozen portion of the extracellular fluid compartment leading to water shifting from the intracellular space to the extracellular space. The water loss induces intracellular dehydration and pH change; this is followed by cell shrinkage and denaturing of cellular proteins. With further drops in temperature, beyond −15 °C, intracellular crystallization takes place and cell metabolism begins to fail. This leads to mechanical breaks of the cellular membrane and cell apoptosis is induced after the thermal injury. Complete cell death is likely to occur at temperatures lower than −40 °C after two cycles.

Vasodilatation around the targeted tissue occurs after thawing causing hyperpermeability of vessel walls. This leads to endothelial damage and microthrombi formation resulting in regional tissue hypoxia and secondary necrosis of the tissue [19].

Procedure

After induction of adequate general anesthesia, the patient is placed in the lithotomy position. A TRUS probe is inserted per rectum and affixed to a fixation device. A template grid is placed in front of the perineum secured to the fixation device. Two to four cryoprobes are introduced through the perineum under imaging guidance. Catheter warmer is placed per urethra and placed on continuous warmer irrigation. Double freeze-thaw cycles are delivered with the goal of bringing the temperature below −40 °C. Argon and helium gases are used for freezing and thawing, respectively. After the two cycles are completed, the needles are removed and the urethral warmer keep running for 20 additional minutes. The urethra warmer is then removed and a Folcy catheter inserts and left indwelling for 5–7 days. Visualization of the ice ball in real time using ultrasonography allows treating the focal cancer zone, minimizing injury to adjacent structures (Figs. 10.1, 10.2, 10.3, and 10.4).

Current Studies: Oncologic and Functional Outcomes

Cryotherapy is the most studied ablative therapy. Onik et al. were first to report outcomes of FT in 2002 followed by an update of their experience in 2008. They reported on 48 patients with a mean follow-up of 54 months (range 2–10 years).

Fig. 10.1 Perineal template with inserted cryoprobes to treat right side distal lesion

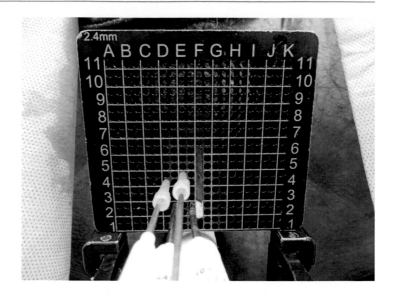

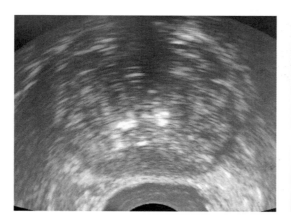

Fig. 10.2 Inserted cryoprobe needles as seen on ultrasound image

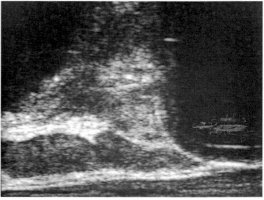

Fig. 10.4 Iceball—sagittal view. Notice sparing of proximal prostate

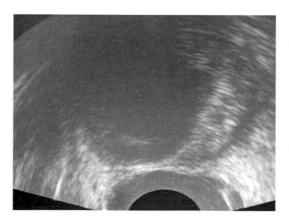

Fig. 10.3 Iceball—transverse view

Ninety-four percent had no evidence of cancer according to ASTRO (American Society of Therapeutic Radiology and Oncology) criteria. Potency was maintained in 36 of 40 patients (90 %) and all were continent after treatment [20].

Ellis et al. reported on 60 patients treated with focal cryotherapy. The mean follow-up was 15 months. 84 % of the patients were biochemically disease-free (ASTRO criteria) and 3.6 % reported urinary incontinence [21].

In 2007, Lambert et al. reported on 25 men treated with hemiablation of the gland. Mean follow-up was 28 months. Eighty-four percent had experienced no biochemical failure, defined as

50 % PSA increase over nadir level. Seven patients underwent a repeat biopsy. One patient had prostate cancer in the area of previous cryoablation and 2 patients in the contralateral gland [18].

Bahn et al. reported on 31 patients. Biochemical disease-free rate by ASTRO criteria was 92.8 %. Biopsy in one patient with biochemical recurrence demonstrated cancer at the apex of the untreated side. Potency preservation rate was 88.9 % (40.7 % with PDE-5 inhibitors) [22].

More recently Ward et al. published an update from the Cryo On Line Database (COLD) registry; biochemical disease-free rate was 75.7 % (ASTRO criteria) at 36 months, urinary continence was 98.4 %, and preservation of spontaneous erections 58.1 % [23].

Overall, biochemical disease-free rate is 75–94 % [18, 20–23]. Nevertheless definitions of biochemical recurrence and patient's selection criteria were variable between studies. These studies are limited due to small number of patients and short follow up. The reported functional outcomes are encouraging, with a good potency and urinary continence rates. No other significant morbidities were reported (Table 10.1).

Future Direction

Focal Cryotherapy is a promising treatment option for selected patients with early prostate cancer. Future research should be directed towards establishing better means of characterizing clinically significant disease and developing improved image technologies to target treatment.

High-Intensity Focused Ultrasound

Overview

HIFU was first described in 1995 as a technique to treat localized prostate cancer. Most of the current reports describe whole prostate gland treatments. HIFU can also be used for focal tumor ablation with the goal of sparing normal gland and minimizing the adverse effects of whole gland treatment. There are currently two devices available for treatment: The Ablatherm HIFU device (EDAP S.A., Lyon, France) and The Sonable 500 (Focus surgery, IN, USA). Both devices are widely used in Europe, Canada, and Japan. HIFU is still considered investigational in the United States and is not currently approved by the Federal Drugs Administration (FDA). Several trials are currently in progress to establish the efficacy and safety of HIFU.

Mechanism of Action

During HIFU ultrasound waves are emitted from a transducer and absorbed in the target area inducing necrosis. Two main mechanisms are involved in the HIFU ablation effect: A thermal effect is heat generation due to absorption of the acoustic energy with a rapid elevation of temperature in the targeted tissues, which denatures proteins, destroys lipid-based membranes, and finally results in instantaneous and irreversible coagulative necrosis. This is the primary mechanism for

Table 10.1 Summarizes oncologic and functional outcomes of focal cryotherapy

Name	N	Mean follow-up (months)	BR criteria	BDF (%)	Potency (%)	Continence (%)
Onik [20]	48	54	ASTRO	94	90	100
Ellis [21]	60	15	ASTRO	80.4	–	96.4
Lambert [18]	25	28	PSA nadir + 50 %	84	71	–
Bahn [22]	31	70	ASTRO	92.8	89	–
Ward [23]	1,160	36	ASTRO	75.7	58.1	98.4

American society for therapeutic radiology and oncology consensus panel. Int J Radiat Oncol Biol Phys. 1997;37:1035–41.
ASTRO American Society for Therapeutic Radiology and Oncology, *BR* biochemical recurrence, *BDF* biochemical disease-free

tumor cell destruction. The mechanical effect leads to cavitation causing additional damage to the prostate and periprostatic tissue. The treatment area is heated for 3 s and cooled for 6 s using real-time images. Surrounding tissue is minimally affected as the energy decreases sharply outside the target zone [24–26].

Procedure

Ablatherm® after induction of general anesthesia, the patient lies on his left side, thighs, and legs flexed 90° on the trunk. A transrectal HIFU probe is inserted per rectum. The probe delivers a beam of high-focused convergent ultrasounds, causing heat and tissue destruction. The ultrasound beam absorption creates an immediate increase in temperature (85–100 °C). The treatment is performed using contiguous HIFU shots 1.8 mm apart with 4-s shot duration and a 12-s interval between shots. At the end of the procedure an 18 F Foley catheter is placed for 1–2 weeks.

Sonablate® 500 after induction of general anesthesia, the patient is placed in the lithotomy position and HIFU probe is introduced per rectum. Treatment is monitored with real-time TRUS. After the procedure, an 18 F Foley catheter is placed and left for 1–2 weeks.

Current Studies, Oncologic, and Functional Outcomes

In 2008, Muto et al. reported on 29 patients who underwent transrectal HIFU (Sonablate 500). Two years biochemical disease-free rates by ASTRO criteria in patients with low and intermediate risk prostate cancer were 83.3 % and 53.6 % respectively [25].

Ahmed et al. reported a prospective study phase I/II trial in 20 men with prostate cancer who underwent a transrectal hemiablation of the prostate with the Sonablate 500 device. Patients were divided into low ($n=5$) and intermediate risk ($n=15$). Follow-up included MRI; TRUS-guided biopsies and PSA measurement at 1 month after the procedure and every 3 months thereafter. There was no histological evidence of cancer in 89 % of

treated lobe. A trifecta status (pad-free, leak-free continence, erections sufficient for intercourse and cancer control) was achieved in 89 % at 12 months [26]. Ahmed et al. reported their results on 41 men treated between 2007 and 2010; using the Sonable 500 device and who were diagnosed by a combination of multiparametric MRI and Transperineal Template Mapping Biopsies (TTMP). Follow-up was scheduled every 3 months after treatment. Questioners were used to assess potency and incontinence. Eighty-nine percent (31 of 35 patients) described erections sufficient for penetration at 12 months. Fourteen required phosphodiestrerase-5 inhibitors. Of 38 men with no urinary leak at baseline 100 % were leak-free by 9 months. Thirty-nine of 41 patients underwent postoperative biopsy. Nine (23 %) had evidence of cancer. MRI at 6 months showed residual cancer in the treated areas in nine men; seven of whom had cancer confirmed on biopsy. Of those with positive biopsies, four patients underwent retreatment and none showed significant disease at 12 months on MRI [27]. These studies demonstrate good morbidity outcomes and promising cancer control rates. Limitations to these studies included small number of patients and short-term follow-up. Some authors considered hemiablation as a focal therapy with no consensus on definition regardless of grade, volume, or location of the tumor. Hemiablation may represent overtreatment since low-volume and low-grade lesions may be treated with more focused therapy.

Future Direction

Additional studies and more conclusive findings are needed. Trials are currently ongoing (NCT01194648, NCT00988130, NCT00987675) to establish the safety and efficacy of HIFU.

Photodynamic Therapy

Overview

The first report describing PDT for prostate cancer with light-sensitive agent using a transurethral approach was published in 1990 [28].

PDT is an experimental ablative technology which employs photosensitizing properties selectively taken up by prostate cancer cells and produces free oxygen radicals upon exposure to light of a specific wavelength which results in the destruction of the tissue.

As photosensitizers accumulate in some organs including skin and eyes, patients require light protection until the photosensitizer is no longer present. PDT is theoretically more tissue-specific and could preserve neurovascular bundle better than other FT. Recent advances in PDT have led to improvements of the synthesis of new-generation photosensitizers with better stability, shorter half-lives, and faster metabolism. The rapid clearance of these new agents from the circulation could avoid prolonged photosensitivity. Vascular photodynamic therapy (VTP) utilizes more recent photosensitizers derived from chlorophyll, such as WST09 (Tookad), to induce vascular damage leading to thrombosis and necrosis of the target tissue [29, 30].

Mechanism of Action

A Photosensitizer is injected intravenously and is distributed throughout the body; during treatment, small energy-delivering probes are placed in the prostate through optical fibers that deliver low power laser light to activate the administered drug. VTP usually uses WST09 that absorbs light near to infrared wavelength with maximum light energy absorption at 763 nm. This long light absorption wavelength allows deeper light penetration into tissues. The photosensitizer enhances sensitivity of the tumor vasculature to light energy. Damage to the vascular endothelium is followed by platelet aggregation and vascular coagulation around the tip of the fiber with subsequent localized tissue necrosis.

Procedure

The photosensitizer is given intravenously and accumulates in prostate tissue. The drug is then activated 2–5 days later by light of a specific

wavelength from laser. Drug dose and light doses are variable and most are still under investigation. Manipulation of drug and light can result in varied volumes of ablation. A transperineal approach, using a brachytherapy template, guides insertion of optical fibers that deliver low power laser light.

Currents Studies and Future Direction

Few studies have been published regarding PDT. Trial NCT01310894 is currently under way to evaluate this treatment modality. PDT research focuses on determining the optimal type and dose of photosensitizing agent as well as the optimal light exposure time for treatment.

Focal Laser Ablation

Overview

A new source of energy that applied for FT is Laser Ablation (FLA). Low-power laser delivers luminous energy guided by real-time imaging; FLA produces a coagulative necrosis zone within a controlled area, reducing the risk of damaging adjacent structures.

Mechanism of Action

FLA is based on a photothermal effect which results from the absorption of radiant energy by tissue-receptive chromophores, which induces heat energy in a very short time. Increased temperature may cause irreversible damages and tissue destruction. The thermal effect depends on the amount of heat energy delivered but also on the depth of light distribution. For this reason, deep tissue damage is dependent on the wavelength of the laser used, usually a range between 590 and 1,064 nm. The extension of thermal tissue damage depends on both temperature and duration. Irreversible protein denaturation will occur around 60 °C, while over 60 °C, coagulation is quasi-instantaneous. Macroscopic appearance of coagulation areas of FLA corresponds to well-demarcated foci of necrosis surrounded by a small rim of hemorrhage with no viable glandular tissue after vital staining, based on immunoreactivity with cytokeratin [31, 32].

Procedure

The patient is placed under general anesthesia and in dorsal lithotomy position. A 2-way urethral catheter is inserted at the beginning of the procedure. A modified brachytherapy template is used for transperineal placement of the laser fibers. Depending on the size of the planned treatment volume, 1 or 2 fibers will be used. Wavelengths in the range of 590–1,064 nm are the most adequate to induce photothermal effect. An optimal fiber location is monitored with real-time ultrasound or other imaging modalities.

Currents Studies and Future Direction

There is currently very limited data available for FLA. Lindner et al. reported a pilot study in 4 patients, addressing feasibility. They correlated MRI findings with histopathology after radical prostatectomy (RP). No viable cells were found in treated regions and MRI findings correlated well with pathology reports [33]. The same group also reported their findings on image-guided focal laser ablation in 12 patients. Six patients (50 %) had negative biopsies 3–6 months following treatment and 67 % were free of tumor in targeted area. No relevant morbidities were reported [34]. Larger trials are currently in progress (NCT00805883, NCT01377753) addressing feasibility. Laser technology is improving and may lead to better focal therapy.

Conclusion

Early detection of prostate cancer has led to over-diagnosis of clinically insignificant tumors. We currently lack reliable tools to select optimal candidates for definitive treatment. With improved diagnostic modalities and optimal focal therapies the rate of complications may be markedly diminished with excellent cancer control. Men diagnosed with low-risk disease will continue to seek treatment despite excellent outcomes with active surveillance in appropriately selected patients. Researchers continue to develop new approaches to treat low-grade prostate cancer while minimizing side effects. Focal Therapy is emerging as a new treatment modality that could provide a bridge between active surveillance and more aggressive treatments for patients with low-risk tumors, achieving cancer control while minimizing morbidity. Several energy sources are being tested for this indication. The available literature is limited regarding focal therapies. Most evidence is derived from case series and small phase I trials. Ablative modalities such as VTP and FLA have only demonstrated technical feasibility to date. To make this approach valid, further research to establish patient selection criteria, new and more accurate imaging parameters, and regular follow-up protocols are needed. It is expected that new energy source will be introduced in the near future for focal therapy.

References

1. American Cancer Society. Cancer facts and figures 2012. Atlanta, GA: American Cancer Society; 2012.
2. Borofsky MS, Ito T, Rosenkrantz AB, et al. Focal therapy for prostate cancer—where are we in 2011? Ther Adv Urol. 2011;3(4):183–92.
3. Wilt TJ, MacDonald R, Rutks I, et al. Systematic review: comparative effectiveness and harms of treatment for clinically localized prostate cancer. Ann Inter Med. 2008;148:435–48.
4. Crawford ED, Barqawi A. Targeted focal therapy: a minimally invasive ablation technique for early prostate cancer. Oncology. 2007;21(1):27–32.
5. Scattoni V, Zlotta A, Montironi R, et al. Extended and saturation prostatic biopsy in the diagnosis and characterization of prostate cancer: a critical analysis of the literature. Eur Urol. 2007;52:1309–22.
6. Onik G, Miessau M, Bostwick DG. Three-dimensional prostate mapping biopsy has a potentially significant impact on prostate cancer management. J Clin Oncol. 2009;27(26):4321–6.
7. Djavan B, Susani M, Bursa B, et al. Predictability and significance of multifocal prostate cancer in the radical prostatectomy specimen. Tech Urol. 1999;5(3):139–42.

8. Karavitakis M, Winkler M, Abel P, et al. Histological characteristics of the index lesion in whole-mount radical prostatectomy specimens: implications for focal therapy. Prostate Cancer Prostatic Dis. 2011; 14(1):46–52.

9. Noguchi M, Stamey TA, Mcneal JE, et al. Prognostic factors for multifocal prostate cancer in radical prostatectomy specimens: lack of significance of secondary cancers. J Urol. 2003;170:459–63.

10. Eggener SE, Scardino PT, Carroll PR, et al. Focal therapy for localized prostate cancer: a critical appraisal of rationale and modalities. J Urol. 2007; 178(6):2260–7.

11. de la Rosette J, Ahmed H, Barentsz J, et al. Focal therapy in prostate cancer-report from a consensus panel. J Endourol. 2010;24(5):775–80.

12. Lindner U, Trachtenberg J. Focal therapy for localized prostate cancer-choosing the middle ground. Can Urol Assoc J. 2009;3(4):333–5.

13. Dickinson L, Ahmed HU, Allen C, et al. Magnetic resonance imaging for the detection, localisation, and characterization of prostate cancer: recommendations from a European consensus meeting. Eur Urol. 2011;59(4):477–94.

14. Ouzzane A, Puech P, Lemaitre L, et al. Combined multiparametric MRI and targeted biopsies improve anterior prostate cancer detection, staging, and grading. Urology. 2011;78(6):1356–62.

15. Puech P, Potiron E, Lemaitre L, et al. Dynamic contrastenhanced-magnetic resonance imaging evaluation of intraprostatic prostate cancer: correlation with radical prostatectomy specimens. Urology. 2009;74(5):1094–9.

16. Onik G, Barzell W. Transperineal 3D mapping biopsy of the prostate: an essential tool in selecting patients for focal prostate cancer therapy. Urol Oncol. 2008;26(5):506–10.

17. Barqawi AB, Rove KO, Gholizadeh S, et al. The role of 3-dimensional mapping biopsy in decision making for treatment of apparent early stage prostate cancer. J Urol. 2011;186(1):80–5.

18. Lambert EH, Bolte K, Masson P, et al. Focal cryosurgery: encouraging health outcomes for unifocal prostate cancer. Urology. 2007;69(6):1117–20.

19. Babaian RJ, Donnelly B, Bahn D, et al. Best practice statement on cryosurgery for the treatment of localized prostate cancer. J Urol. 2008;180:1993–2004.

20. Onik G, Vaughan D, Lotenfoe R, et al. The "male lumpectomy": focal therapy for prostate cancer using cryoablation results in 48 patients with at least 2-year follow-up. Urol Oncol. 2008;26(5):500–5.

21. Ellis DS, Manny Jr TB, Rewcastle JC. Focal cryosurgery followed by penile rehabilitation as primary treatment for localized prostate cancer: initial results. Urology. 2007;70:9–15.

22. Bahn DK, Silverman P, Lee F, et al. Focal prostate cryoablation: initial results show cancer control and potency preservation. J Endourol. 2006;20(9): 688–92.

23. Ward JF, Jones JS. Focal cryotherapy for localized prostate cancer: a report from the national Cryo On-Line Database (COLD) Registry. BJU Int. 2012;109(11):1648–54.

24. Maestroni U, Ziveri M, Azzolini N, et al. High intensity focused ultrasound (HIFU): a useful alternative choice in prostate cancer treatment. Preliminary results. Acta Biomed. 2008;79(3):211–6.

25. Muto S, Yoshii T, Saito K, et al. Focal therapy with high-intensity-focused ultrasound in the treatment of localized prostate cancer. Japan J Clin Oncol. 2008;38(3):192–9.

26. Ahmed HU, Freeman A, Kirkham A, et al. Focal therapy for localized prostate cancer: a phase I/II trial. J Urol. 2011;185(4):1246–54.

27. Ahmed HU, Hindley RG, Dickinson L, et al. Focal therapy for localised unifocal and multifocal prostate cancer: a prospective development study. Lancet Oncol. 2012;13(6):622–32.

28. Windahl T, Andersson SO, Lofgren L. Photodynamic therapy of localized prostatic cancer. Lancet. 1990; 336:1139.

29. Arumainayagam N, Moore CM, Ahmed HU, et al. Photodynamic therapy for focal ablation of the prostate. World J Urol. 2010;28(5):571–6.

30. Moore C, Pendse D, Emberton M. Photodynamic therapy for prostate cancer a review of current status and future promise. Nat Clin Pract Urol. 2009;6(1): 18–30.

31. Lindner U, Lawrentschuk N, Trachtenberg J. Focal laser ablation for localized prostate cancer. J Endourol. 2010;24(5):791–7.

32. Colin P, Mordon S, Nevoux P, et al. Focal laser ablation of prostate cancer: definition, needs, and future. Adv Urol. 2012;2012:589160.

33. Lindner U, Lawrentschuk N, Weersink R, et al. Focal laser ablation for prostate cancer followed by radical prostatectomy: validation of focal therapy and imaging accuracy. Eur Urol. 2010;57(6):1111–4.

34. Lindner U, Weersink RA, Haider MA, et al. Image guided photothermal focal therapy for localized prostate cancer: phase I trial. J Urol. 2009;182(4): 1371–7.

Index

R.V. Khanna et al. (eds.), *Surgical Techniques for Prostate Cancer*,
DOI 10.1007/978-1-4939-1616-0, © Springer Science+Business Media New York 2015